Scars: Prevention, Correction, and Reduction

Guest Editor

STEVEN ROSS MOBLEY, MD

FACIAL PLASTIC SURGERY CLINICS OF NORTH AMERICA

www.facialplastic.theclinics.com

August 2011 • Volume 19 • Number 3

SAUNDERS an imprint of ELSEVIER, Inc.

W.B. SAUNDERS COMPANY
A Division of Elsevier Inc.

1600 John F. Kennedy Blvd., Suite 1800, Philadelphia, PA 19103-2899

http://www.theclinics.com

FACIAL PLASTIC SURGERY CLINICS OF NORTH AMERICA Volume 19, Number 3
August 2011 ISSN 1064-7406, ISBN 978-1-4557-0443-9

Editor: Joanne Husovski

Facial Plastic Surgery Clinics of North America (ISSN 1064-7406) is published quarterly by Elsevier Inc., 360 Park Avenue South, New York, NY 10010-1710. Months of issue are February, May, August, and November. Business and Editorial Offices: 1600 John F. Kennedy Blvd., Suite 1800, Philadelphia, PA 19103-2899. Periodicals postage paid at New York, NY, and additional mailing offices. Subscription prices are $329.00 per year (US individuals), $459.00 per year (US institutions), $375.00 per year (Canadian individuals), $550.00 per year (Canadian institutions), $449.00 per year (foreign individuals), $550.00 per year (foreign institutions), $156.00 per year (US students), and $217.00 per year (foreign students). Foreign air speed delivery is included in all *Clinics* subscription prices. All prices are subject to change without notice. POSTMASTER: Send address changes to *Facial Plastic Surgery Clinics*, Elsevier Health Sciences Division, Subscription Customer Service, 3251 Riverport Lane, Maryland Heights, MO 63043. **Customer service: 1-800-654-2452 (US and Canada); 1-314-447-8871 (outside US and Canada); Fax: 314-447-8029; E-mail:journalscustomerservice-usa@elsevier.com (for print support); journalsonline support-usa@elsevier.com (for online support).**

Reprints. For copies of 100 or more of articles in this publication, please contact the Commercial Reprints Department, Elsevier Inc., 360 Park Avenue South, New York, NY 10010-1710. Tel.: 212-633-3812; Fax: 212-462-1935; E-mail: reprints@elsevier.com.

Facial Plastic Surgery Clinics of North America is covered in *MEDLINE/PubMed* (*Index Medicus*).

Printed and bound by CPI Group (UK) Ltd, Croydon, CR0 4YY

Transferred to Digital Print 2011

Contributors

CONSULTING EDITOR

J. REGAN THOMAS, MD, FACS
Professor and Chairman, Department
of Otolaryngology, University of Illinois
at Chicago, Chicago, Illinois

EDITORIAL BOARD

SHAN R. BAKER, MD
Professor and Chief, Section of Plastic
and Reconstructive Surgery, University
of Michigan, Ann Arbor, Michigan

ROBERT KELLMAN, MD
Professor and Chairman, Department
of Otolaryngology, State University of
New York Upstate Medical University,
Syracuse, New York

RUSSELL W.H. KRIDEL, MD
Clinical Associate Professor, Department
of Otolaryngology–Head and Neck Surgery,
Division of Facial Plastic Surgery, University of
Texas Health Science Center, Houston, Texas

STEPHEN W. PERKINS, MD
Private Practitioner, Perkins Facial Plastic
Surgery, Indianapolis, Indiana

ANTHONY P. SCLAFANI, MD, FACS
Director of Facial Plastic Surgery,
The New York Eye and Ear Infirmary,
New York, New York; and Professor of
Otolaryngology–Head and Neck Surgery,
New York Medical College, Valhalla,
New York

GUEST EDITOR

STEVEN ROSS MOBLEY, MD
Associate Professor, Director of Facial Plastic
Surgery, Division of Otolaryngology–Head and
Neck Surgery, University of Utah Health
Sciences Center, School of Medicine,
Salt Lake City, Utah

AUTHORS

TINA S. ALSTER, MD
Washington Institute of Dermatologic Laser
Surgery, Washington, DC

LUCY BARR, MD
Barr Facial Plastic Surgery, Salt Lake City, Utah

ALFONSO BARRERA, MD, FACS
Clinical Assistant Professor of Plastic Surgery,
Baylor College of Medicine, Plastic and
Cosmetic Surgery, Houston, Texas

JENNIFER R. DECKER, MD
Resident Physician, Department of
Otolaryngology–Head and Neck Surgery,
Northwestern University Feinberg School of
Medicine, McGaw Medical Center, Chicago,
Illinois

RICHARD FITZPATRICK, MD
Cosmetic Laser Dermatology, San Diego,
California

CHONG WEE FOO, MD
Resident, Department of Dermatology,
University of Utah, Salt Lake City, Utah

ERIC A. GANTWERKER, MS, MD
Resident Physician, Department of
Otolaryngology–Head and Neck Surgery,
University of Cincinnati and Cincinnati
Children's Hospital Medical Center,
Cincinnati, Ohio

DAVID B. HOM, MD, FACS
Professor, Division of Facial Plastic and
Reconstructive Surgery, Department of
Otolaryngology–Head and Neck Surgery,
University of Cincinnati and Cincinnati
Children's Hospital Medical Center,
Cincinnati, Ohio

HAENA KIM, MD
Resident Physician, Department of
Otolaryngology–Head and Neck Surgery,
McGaw Medical Center, Northwestern
University Feinberg School of Medicine,
Chicago, Illinois

STEVEN ROSS MOBLEY, MD
Associate Professor, Director of Facial Plastic
Surgery, Division of Otolaryngology–Head and
Neck Surgery, University of Utah Health
Sciences Center, School of Medicine,
Salt Lake City, Utah

J. STUART NELSON, MD, PhD
Beckman Laser Institute, University of
California, Irvine, California

SEPEHR OLIAEI, MD
Beckman Laser Institute, University of
California, Irvine; Division of Facial Plastic
Surgery, Department of Otolaryngology–Head
and Neck Surgery, University of California,
Irvine, Orange, California

KRISHNA G. PATEL, MD, PhD
Assistant Professor, Director of Facial Plastic
and Reconstructive Surgery, Department of
Otolaryngology–Head and Neck Surgery,
Medical University of South Carolina,
Charleston, South Carolina

GEOFFREY B. PITZER, MD
Otolaryngology Resident, Department of
Otolaryngology–Head and Neck Surgery,
Medical University of South Carolina,
Charleston, South Carolina

NATHAN TODD NELSON SCHREIBER, MD
Otolaryngology Resident, Division of
Otolaryngology–Head and Neck Surgery,
University of Utah Health Sciences Center,
School of Medicine, Salt Lake City, Utah

WILLIAM W. SHOCKLEY, MD, FACS
W. Paul Biggers Distinguished Professor,
Chief, Facial Plastic and Reconstructive
Surgery, Department of Otolaryngology–
Head and Neck Surgery, University of
North Carolina School of Medicine,
Chapel Hill, North Carolina

DOUGLAS M. SIDLE, MD, FACS
Director, Assistant Professor, Division
of Facial Plastic Surgery, Department of
Otolaryngology–Head and Neck Surgery,
Northwestern University Feinberg School of
Medicine, Northwestern Memorial Hospital,
Chicago, Illinois

JOSEPH F. SOBANKO, MD
Assistant Professor of Dermatology, Perelman
Center for Advanced Medicine, University of
Pennsylvania, Philadelphia, Pennsylvania

JOSHUA B. SUROWITZ, MD
Department of Otolaryngology–Head and Neck
Surgery, University of North Carolina at
Chapel Hill, Chapel Hill, North Carolina

PAYAM TRISTANI-FIROUZI, MD
Assistant Professor of Dermatology,
Department of Dermatology, University
of Utah, Salt Lake City, Utah

BRIAN J. WONG, MD, PhD
Beckman Laser Institute, University of
California, Irvine; Division of Facial Plastic
Surgery, Department of Otolaryngology–Head
and Neck Surgery, University of California,
Irvine, Orange, California

Contents

It is important to understand the histology and physiology of skin for the prediction and optimization of wound healing. Optimal postoperative wound healing to minimize scarring entails minimizing local, systemic, and environmental factors that lead to poor wound healing. Keeping the wound clean and moist, minimizing trauma, and infection are the local wound tenets. Systemic tenets include minimizing medications that inhibit processes of wound healing, maintaining adequate nutrition, pain palliation, UV protection, and smoking cessation. This article presents the dynamic process of wound healing and the basic tenets to minimize scarring.

This article addresses the use of scar revision surgery as it relates to the use of Z-plasty, W-plasty, and geometric broken line closure. Each of these techniques is discussed in detail and the author provides perspectives regarding the indications, advantages, and limitations of each procedure. The surgeon should be experienced with each of these and apply these methods as appropriate. As with any technique, careful preoperative planning along with meticulous execution will lead to optimal results.

Nasal reconstruction is one of the most challenging aspects of facial plastic surgery. The authors present reconstructive techniques to maximize the final aesthetic result and minimize scarring. They discuss techniques used in nasal reconstruction with a paramedian forehead flap (PMFF) that help to achieve these goals and minimize the chance of complications, including performing a surgical delay, using generous, supportive cartilage grafts, adding extra length and bulk to the flap at the alar rim and using topical nitroglycerin and triamcinolone injections when indicated. The steps outlined can help to create a more elegant and consistent result in PMFF nasal reconstruction.

Scars after facial trauma or surgery can be a source of distress for patients, and facial plastic surgeons are frequently called upon to help manage them. Although no technique can remove a scar, numerous treatment modalities have been developed to improve facial scar appearance with varying levels of invasiveness. This article reviews techniques that camouflage scars without surgical intervention. Topical scar treatments, camouflage cosmetics, use of hairstyling and glasses, and facial prosthetics are discussed. In addition, professional counseling is provided on selection and application of topical cosmetics for use as part of an office practice.

Proper wound care has broad applications for all clinicians. Much of the future direction for enhancing wound repair focuses on key cells and growth factors, which is why possessing a strong understanding of the basic physiology of wound healing is imperative. This article first provides a thorough review of the phases of wound healing followed by a discussion on the latest wound management strategies. Wound conditions and surgical techniques are important components for optimizing wound healing and preventing complications. Special consideration has been given to the unique settings of contaminated wounds, open wounds, or avulsed tissue.

Keloids result from an abnormal wound-healing process in which the normal regulatory pathways during tissue regeneration and scar remodeling are disrupted. While the pathogenesis of keloids continues to be investigated, numerous treatment options exist. Although prevention of keloid formation is the best management, early recognition of keloid formation is integral in treatment and prevention of recurrence. Surgical resection with adjuvant silicone gel sheeting or triamcinolone injection is common, but can still result in recurrence. New treatments include chemotherapeutics such as 5-fluorouracil, bleomycin, and mitomycin C. Although further clinical investigation is required for newer treatments, initial results are promising.

This article describes the physiology of wound healing, discusses considerations and techniques for dermabrasion, and presents case studies and figures for a series of patients who underwent dermabrasion after surgeries for facial trauma.

Cutaneous injuries that result in scar formation are relatively common, leading patients to seek treatment for cosmetic or functional improvement. Treatments that have the potential to improve or eliminate scarring include radiation therapy, surgical excision, and intralesional injections of corticosteroids, 5-flourouracil, or bleomycin. Unfortunately, these methods are associated with high recurrence rates and untoward sequelae such as skin atrophy, dyspigmentation, and pain. Laser scar revision is a safe procedure with clinically demonstrable efficacy and minimal side effects when used alone or in combination with other scar treatments. The specifics of current laser scar revision techniques are addressed in this overview.

This article is a clinically practical review structured around the specific applications of laser technologies used in acute management of soft tissue injuries in surgical incisions and trauma. Surgical and traumatic incisions and injuries provide the clinician with the unique opportunity to follow the progression and maturation of the wound healing response from a very early stage. There has been a recent interest in early cosmetic optimization of surgical and traumatic wounds on the face using optical technologies. Early clinical results for acute laser intervention starting immediately after suture removal or the first several weeks after repair have been very promising.

There is no universally accepted treatment regimen and no evidence-based literature to guide management of hypertrophic scars. This article summarizes the existing literature regarding topical treatments such as silicone gel sheeting and ointment, onion extract, vitamin E, pressure garment therapy, massage therapy, and topical imiquimod 5% cream in the management of hypertrophic scars.

Loss of hair-bearing tissue in the head and neck area can result from surgery, trauma, burns, tumors, and infection, as well as a diversity of inflammatory conditions, and the resulting defect can present a challenging problem for the reconstructive surgeon. Hair transplantation can be used as a reconstructive method alone or in conjunction with other techniques. The current method of using follicular unit grafts has led to natural restorations for a variety of areas including not only the scalp but also eyebrows, eyelashes, and beard areas. Camouflage provided by hair grafts can provide restoration not obtainable with other methods.

Facial Plastic Surgery Clinics of North America

THE CLINICS ARE NOW AVAILABLE ONLINE!

Access your subscription at:
www.theclinics.com

Scars: Clinical Evidence Base and Patient Impact

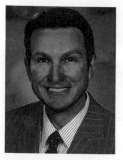

Steven Ross Mobley, MD
Guest Editor

As Facial Plastic Surgeons, we are trained to evaluate scars in terms of clinical variables. Are they flat? Are they wide? Are they in parallel to relaxed skin tension lines? For many patients, though, the potential impact of scars is far greater than simple, measurable assessments, and that effect is much more difficult to assess.

As an example from my own life, I have had a premalignant lesion removed from my cheek. I left the dermatologist's office with a small circular bandage over the repair site. While this adhesive bandage was probably no more than one inch in diameter, I still remember being stared at by complete strangers in the halls of the hospital, each of them seeming to wonder, "What happened to him?" I was experiencing firsthand how the treatment of this small facial lesion was altering the way in which I normally interacted with other people. This admittedly minor experience nevertheless gave me pause and has helped me to have better empathy for all facial reconstruction patients.

At times, doctors may forget the profound impact a facial scar can have on a patient's self-perception. I have treated a patient with 70% burns from mining slag who seemed to be unaffected by what any casual observer would consider a completely disfiguring facial injury. I have also treated a very attractive 55-year-old female who had lost nearly half her nose and underwent a near-flawless reconstruction with a paramedian forehead flap. For this woman, however, her experience with facial scarring marked the beginning of her life into a downward spiral. For her, no longer being "perfectly" beautiful was too great a burden to bear. She lost her family and her career as a result of depression and feeling incapable of interacting in public. While most people would say she had an excellent surgical result, for her, things would never be the same.

I thank each author for their excellent contributions to this *Facial Plastic Surgery Clinics of North America*. The information within this volume should help each of us to improve our techniques, to follow guidelines established by evidenced-based literature, and, in the final result, to relieve both the physical and the psychosocial burdens of facial scars. As a patient with significant facial scarring once wrote me, "My bark is much worse than my bite. Don't be frightened by first impressions—In my heart I truly am smiling."

As Facial Plastic Surgeons, we must remember that each patient we care for can, and will, have a different reaction to facial scarring. I hope that the articles contained within this *Facial Plastic Surgery Clinics* review will bestow some new knowledge on surgeons across the country. If just one surgeon is able to improve his or her practice by implementing a few of the "pearls" included here, then the efforts and contributions of the authors of this volume will have been worth it.

Steven Ross Mobley, MD
Division of Otolaryngology–Head and Neck Surgery
University of Utah Health Sciences Center
50 North Medical Drive
School of Medicine 3C120
Salt Lake City, UT 84132, USA

E-mail address:
steven.mobley@hsc.utah.edu

Facial Plast Surg Clin N Am 19 (2011) ix
doi:10.1016/j.fsc.2011.06.011
1064-7406/11/$ – see front matter

Skin: Histology and Physiology of Wound Healing

Eric A. Gantwerker, MS, MD[a], David B. Hom, MD[b],*

KEYWORDS

- Scarring • Scars • Facial • Wounds • Healing
- Skin histology

Key Points

1. Skin is composed of several layers that are essential to its function and response to injury: the epidermis, dermis, and hypodermis. Healing is a dynamic progression encompassing hemostasis, inflammation, proliferation, and remodeling

2. Pilosebaceous units are the source of all epithelial stem cells essential for reepithelialization and wound healing

3. Multiple extrinsic and intrinsic factors affect healing, specifically the effect of immune system modulation (medications and diseased states)

4. It is most optimal to wait at least 4–6 weeks after smoking cessation for elective surgical interventions

5. Keloids and hypertrophic scarring are a result of overabundant collagen production, and decrease collagen breakdown. Keloids are difficult to treat, due to their recurrent nature. It is important to identify individuals prone to keloid formation for surgical planning purposes

Self-Test Questions

The following questions are intended for the reader to self-test. The answers, with full background, are covered within this article.

The correct answers are provided at the conclusion of the article.

1. A 19-year-old woman is on isotretinoin (Accutane) for acne and has a facial acne scar that she wishes to be dermabraded. What do you counsel the patient about?
   a. She needs to be off the medication for 1 year to limit the risk of scarring
   b. She should continue the medication because the extra vitamin A will improve her healing
   c. You cannot resurface her acne scar because of the long-lasting effects of this medication
   d. Encourage 2 g of vitamin C daily for 2 weeks before the procedure

2. A 73-year-old insulin-dependent diabetic man with a serum glucose level of 300 mmol/L comes to your office for a rhytidectomy. How do you optimize your results?
   a. Refer to endocrinologist for tight diabetic control before surgery
   b. Decline the surgery because the risk of failure is increased
   c. Start the patient on vitamin E supplementation 2000 IE daily 2 weeks before surgery
   d. Double his insulin dose on the morning of his surgery

3. A 30-year-old man has a partial-thickness 4 × 4-cm abrasion on his right cheek. What should be the best treatment?

Disclosures: There are no affiliations, conflicts of interest, or financial disclosures by either author.
[a] Department of Otolaryngology – Head and Neck Surgery, University of Cincinnati and Cincinnati Children's Hospital Medical Center, 231 Albert Sabin Way, Cincinnati, OH, USA
[b] Division of Facial Plastic and Reconstructive Surgery, Department of Otolaryngology – Head and Neck Surgery, University of Cincinnati and Cincinnati Children's Hospital Medical Center, 231 Albert Sabin Way, PO Box 670528, Cincinnati, OH 45267-0528, USA
* Corresponding author.
E-mail address: david.hom@uc.edu

Facial Plast Surg Clin N Am 19 (2011) 441–453
doi:10.1016/j.fsc.2011.06.009
1064-7406/11/$ – see front matter © 2011 Elsevier Inc. All rights reserved.

a. Place a split-thickness skin graft
b. Place a full-thickness skin graft
c. Keep the wound bed moist with a moisture retentive ointment
d. Keep the wound dry to maximize reepithelialization.

4. A 50-year-old man sees you about a large wide scar on his neck. On inquiring, the patient states he had a lymph node removed last year and this scar has grown bigger than the cyst was. What do you counsel him about?
   a. That he most likely has a hypertrophic scar and that the likelihood is that this will not happen on further surgical procedures
   b. That this is a keloid and that with vitamin E ointments it should resolve
   c. That this is a hypertrophic scar that will completely go away with simple excision
   d. That this is a keloid and that multiple procedures along with steroid injections may be required to excise it, but still there is no guarantee it will be removed completely.

The study and treatment of wounds go back to Ancient Egypt. In Ancient Egypt the clean edges of wounds were brought together with tape or stitches and a piece of meat was placed on the wound for the first day. Salves such as honey and Matricaria oil were used. The antibacterial and antiseptic properties of these compounds were later elucidated. Honey was later found to have mild antibacterial effects in controlling *Pseudomonas* and methicillin-resistant *Staphylococcus aureus*.[1] Other wound dressings and salves have been used throughout history until the advent of germ theory, which revolutionized medicine and made a significant impact on surgery and wound care. Research in the last decade has focused on growth factors and cytokines that control the complex wound-healing cascade. Newer research has focused on modulating these signaling molecules to improve healing and prevent scarring.

Wound healing in this article focuses on:

- Basic histologic characteristics of skin
- Four phases of wound healing
- Brief overview of collagen matrices
- Extrinsic and intrinsic factors that disrupt wound healing
- Scarring and current classifications
- Basic principles of wound care and scar treatment.

Although each surgeon has his or her own techniques, some based on evidence and others based on preferences, there are certain tenets that most agree on. Here the authors cover some of the evidence supporting practices, but in the

absence of definitive research their personal experience is relied upon.

The process of wound healing is a dynamic, complex interplay of cytokines, involving many different cell types. The skin has important immune and protective characteristics and has an amazing ability to heal, invariably with scarring. Scarring is quite variable and is based on many factors, dependent on patient characteristics and overall health (intrinsic) as well as the healing environment (extrinsic). All epithelial tissues in the body, except for bone, heal by scar formation rather than regeneration. The skin is not spared by this. It is important to identify wound-healing problems early to minimize scarring.

To understand the effects of injury and potential for scarring, one must first look at the layered histology and physiology of the largest organ in the body. The skin is separated into an epidermis, dermis, and hypodermis. The epidermis itself has 5 layers or strata from superficial to deep: corneum, lucidum, granulosum, spinosum, and basale (**Fig. 1**). The epidermis has variable thickness,

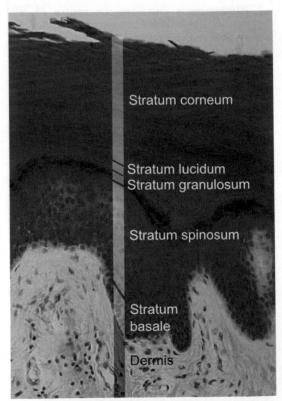

Fig. 1. Histologic section of the epidermis showing the 5 strata from superficial to deep: corneum, lucidum, granulosum, spinosum, and basale. (*Courtesy of* Mikael Haggstrom, Uppsala, Sweden; under GNU Free Documentation License. Available at: http://commons.wikimedia.org/wiki/File:Epidermal_layers.png.)

being thinnest on the eyelids and thickest on the palms and soles.[2,3] This thickness has implications in tissue healing and eventual scarring. The epidermal avascular layer receives its nutrients by diffusion through the dermal layer.

SKIN HISTOLOGY

Keratinocytes make up 95% of the epidermis, and the stratum basale is the source of all replicating keratinocytes. It is these keratinocytes in the basal layer that are primarily responsible for the epidermal response in wound healing.[4] As keratinocytes replicate they push older cells toward the surface, and these cells progressively lose their nucleus and take on a more flattened ovoid shape. This stratified squamous keratinized epithelium undergoes constant turnover, essentially regenerating fully every 48 days. The stratum basale sends down finger-like projections that interdigitate with similar structures reaching up from the dermis. This process forms the rete ridges that are often seen in cross section. Freshly healing wounds as well as skin grafts lack these rete

ridges initially, which makes them susceptible to shear trauma early on.

The epidermis also contains essential appendages including hair follicles with associated sebaceous glands (pilosebaceous unit), eccrine sweat glands, and apocrine glands. The pilosebaceous unit, as well as rete ridges, contains epithelial stem cells that are able to regenerate and differentiate into basal keratinocytes and are essential to the reepithelialization process (**Fig. 2**). These stem cells are critical, as they are relatively undifferentiated, have a large proliferation potential, and have a high capacity for self-renewal.[5] Healing difficulties are seen when these stem cells are destroyed by insults such as burns and even iatrogenic sources such as dermabrasion. When dermabrasion or resurfacing is taken too deep it can destroy the apocrine glands and pilosebaceous unit, leading to improper healing and eventual scarring. Retinoid treatments such as isotretinoin (Accutane) cause atrophy of the sebaceous glands, which is the source of their effectiveness to treat acne. Isotretinoin leads to obvious problems with wound healing, directly reducing the

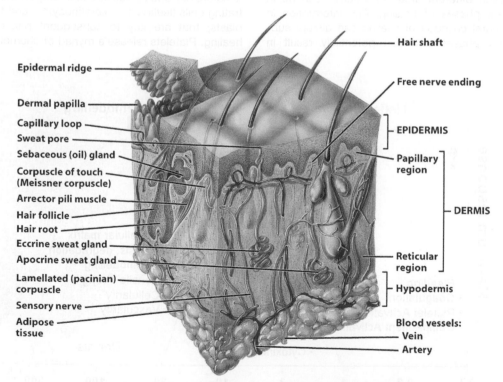

Hair shaft
Epidermal ridge
Dermal papilla
Capillary loop
Sweat pore
Sebaceous (oil) gland
Corpuscle of touch (Meissner corpuscle)
Arrector pili muscle
Hair follicle
Hair root
Eccrine sweat gland
Apocrine sweat gland
Lamellated (pacinian) corpuscle
Sensory nerve
Adipose tissue
Free nerve ending
EPIDERMIS
Papillary region
DERMIS
Reticular region
Hypodermis
Blood vessels:
Vein
Artery

Sectional view of skin and subcutaneous layer

Figure 5-1a Anatomy and Physiology: From Science to Life
© 2006 John Wiley & Sons

Fig. 2. The many appendages of the epidermis and dermis. The pilosebaceous unit is the source of all stem cells essential to the reepithelialization process. (*Reprinted from* Jenkins GW, Tortora GJ, Kemniitz CP. Anatomy and physiology: from science to life. New York: J. Wiley and Sons; 2006. p. 148–71. Chapter: 5; with permission.)

cells needed for reepithelialization. Most surgeons would agree that patients should be off isotretinoin for at least 1 year prior to any surgical resurfacing procedure.[6]

The dermis is the next layer down, which receives the major blood supply for the skin and contains most of the dermal appendages of the skin including the apocrine glands, eccrine glands, and hair follicles. This layer itself is separated into a superficial or papillary dermis and the deeper reticular dermis. As a general rule, any damage that extends into this deeper reticular layer will invariably cause scarring and may require repair with full-thickness grafts or flaps to assure proper healing.

In general there are 4 overlapping phases of wound healing (**Fig. 3**):

1. Hemostasis
2. Inflammation
3. Proliferation
4. Maturation/remodeling.

Although these phases are separated for simplicity reasons they in fact overlap a great deal, and even different areas of wounds can be in different phases of healing. Any interruption in the natural cascade of healing can disrupt subsequent phases and can potentially result in abnormal healing, chronic wounds, and eventual scarring.[4]

Hemostasis

Hemostasis is the initial phase that occurs within seconds to minutes after the initial insult. Initially hemorrhage into the wound exposes platelets to the thrombogenic subendothelium. Platelets are integral to this phase and the entire healing pathway, as they not only serve to provide initial hemostasis but also release multiple cytokines, hormones, and chemokines to set off the remaining phases of healing. Vasoactive substances such as catecholamines and serotonin act via specialized receptors on the endothelium to cause vasoconstriction of the surrounding blood vessels. Smaller vessels are signaled to vasodilate to allow the influx of leukocytes, red blood cells, and plasma proteins. Platelets interact with the GpIIb-IIIa receptor on the collagen of the damaged subendothelium to become activated and form an initial clot. Activated platelets release their granules and ignite the extrinsic and intrinsic coagulation cascades. Fibrin polymerization helps form a mature clot and serves as scaffolding for the infiltrating cells (leukocytes, keratinocytes, and fibroblasts) that are key to subsequent phases of healing. Platelets release a myriad of chemokines

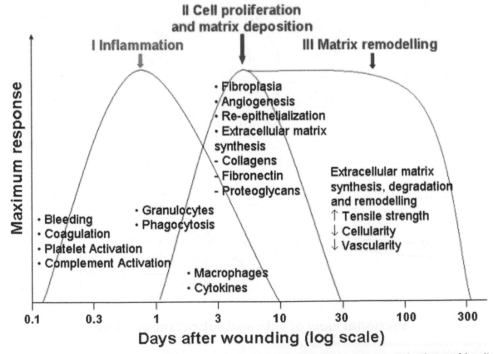

Fig. 3. Time scale of the 4 phases of healing and the many processes that occur at each phase of healing. Any disruption in these processes will ultimately delay healing and lead to scar formation. (*From* Enoch S, Price P. Worldwide Wounds. Available at: http://www.worldwidewounds.com/2004/august/Enoch/Pathophysiology-Of-Healing.html; with permission.)

and cytokines to attract these inflammatory cells to the area. Within minutes, there is an influx of inflammatory cells (predominantly neutrophils and macrophages), leading to the next phase of healing.

Inflammation

The inflammatory phase is heralded by the influx of neutrophils, macrophages, and lymphocytes to the site of injury (**Fig. 4**). Neutrophils are the first leukocytes on site, arriving en masse within the first 24 hours. Neutrophils are soon followed by macrophages, which are attracted by the by-products of neutrophil apoptosis. Phagocytic cells such as macrophages and other lymphocytes appear in the wound to begin to clear debris and bacteria from the wound. These macrophages infiltrate at approximately 48 hours post injury and stay until the conclusion of the inflammatory phase. Macrophages have long been thought to be the key cell to the wound-healing process, and they seem to orchestrate the most important phases of healing. Although they are integral to proper healing, recent research has also looked at their role in improper healing and scarring. Studies of macrophage function have revealed that these key cells are intricate in reepithelialization, granulation tissue formation, angiogenesis, wound cytokine production, and wound contracture.[7] Inflammation is a necessary step of the healing process, and inhibition of this key phase (via anti-inflammatory medications) can result in improper healing. This phase of healing is important to combat infection.[8] If disrupted or prolonged (ie, longer than 3 weeks), this inflammation can lead to a chronic wound, impaired healing, and eventually more scarring. Important factors that can abnormally lengthen this phase of healing include high bacterial load (greater than 10^5 microorganisms per gram of tissue), repeated trauma, and persistent foreign material in the wound.[6] Once the wound has been debrided, the repair or proliferative phase begins.

Proliferation

The proliferative (repair) phase begins early on in the form of reepithelialization (**Fig. 5**). The repair phase also involves capillary budding and extracellular matrix production to fill in the defects left behind from debridement of the wound. Epithelialization is marked by the proliferation and influx of keratinocytes near the leading edge of the wound. As discussed previously, stem cells within the bulbs of the hair follicles and apocrine glands begin to differentiate into keratinocytes and repopulate the stratum basale, and also begin to migrate over the edge of the wound. Once they encounter the mesenchyme of the extracellular matrix (ECM), they attach near the inner wound edge and begin to lay down a new basement membrane. Following this, another row of keratinocytes migrates over the newly laid epithelial cells to fill in the defect. These cells migrate and digest the ECM using proteases until they are in physical contact and they stop migrating, signaled by contact inhibition from neighboring keratinocytes.[9] This reepithelialization protects the wound

Deep wound healing

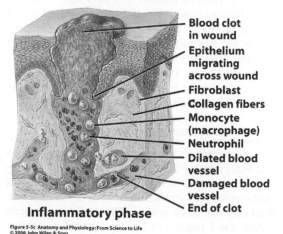

Figure 5-5c Anatomy and Physiology: From Science to Life
© 2006 John Wiley & Sons

Fig. 4. The inflammatory phase heralded by the influx of neutrophils and macrophages into the wound. (*Reprinted from* Jenkins GW, Tortora GJ, Kemniitz CP. Anatomy and physiology: from science to life. New York: J. Wiley and Sons; 2006. p. 148–71. Chapter: 5; with permission.)

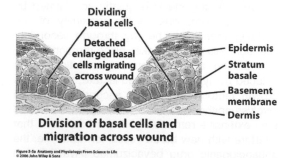

Figure 5-5a Anatomy and Physiology: From Science to Life
© 2006 John Wiley & Sons

Fig. 5. Reepithelialization takes place as keratinocytes differentiate from the stem cells in the basal stratum and migrate over the wound edge to fill in the defect. Migration stops, signaled by contact inhibition as the wound defect fills in. (*Reprinted from* Jenkins GW, Tortora GJ, Kemniitz CP. Anatomy and physiology: from science to life. New York: J. Wiley and Sons; 2006. p. 148–71. Chapter: 5; with permission.)

from infection and desiccation. During this process a layer of uninfected exudates lies over the wound, which provides an important moisture layer and contains growth factors essential to healing. Any improper wound dressings that destroy this healthy layer will result in delayed healing. Underneath this reepithelialization process the ECM continues to be laid down. Wounds healing by secondary intention fill in with granulation tissue. Under the influence of vascular endothelial growth factor (VEGF), angiogenesis begins as the vessels begin to bud from the blood vessels surrounding the wound. Granulation tissue consists of these fibroblasts, new budding vessels, and immature collagen (collagen type III). Some fibroblasts will also begin to differentiate in this phase into myofibroblasts that have contractile function to bring gaping wound edges together.[8]

Angiogenesis/Maturation

Angiogenesis follows a typical pattern of sprouting, looping, and pruning signaled by a complex gradient of cytokines. These small and delicate sprouting vessels repopulate the dermis, and any trauma to this area will lead to destruction of these vessels and delayed healing. Shearing of these new vessels is often a problem in skin grafting, whereby the graft is solely supplied by initial imbibition for 24 hours followed by growth of these vessels into the tissue. It is the role of the bolster placed over these delicate graft sites to prevent hematoma that would limit diffusion of nutrients, but more importantly to prevent shearing of these delicate immature vessels. Bolsters are usually left on for 5 to 7 days to allow these vessels to become more robust and mature, and to resist these shearing forces. Angiogenesis is also a key process affected by primary versus secondary closures. Angiogenesis is greatly accelerated by primary closure, due to the proximity of the budding vessels. In healing through secondary intention, this process takes place through formation of the aforementioned granulation tissue induced by hypoxia, elevated lactate, and various growth factors. Healing by secondary intention involves epithelialization over this granulation and then extensive remodeling. Any medications that interfere with new blood vessel formation (ie, the antiangiogenic drug bevacizumab [Avastin]) can be detrimental to wound healing.

Remodeling

The remodeling phase begins as the provisional ECM and type III collagen is replaced with type I collagen and the remaining cell types of the previous phases undergo apoptosis (**Fig. 6**). With

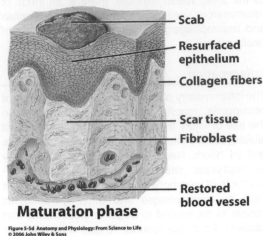

Deep wound healing

- Scab
- Resurfaced epithelium
- Collagen fibers
- Scar tissue
- Fibroblast
- Restored blood vessel

Maturation phase

Figure 5-5d Anatomy and Physiology: From Science to Life
© 2006 John Wiley & Sons

Fig. 6. The maturation phase is longest of the 4 phases and results in the final appearance of the wound. (*Reprinted from* Jenkins GW, Tortora GJ, Kemniitz CP. Anatomy and physiology: from science to life. New York: J. Wiley and Sons; 2006. p. 148–71. Chapter: 5; with permission.)

the laying down of type I collagen, the tensile strength of the wound dramatically increases. Granulation tissue begins to involute and excess blood vessels retract. This phase lasts the longest and results in the final appearance of the wound following healing. A successful remodeling phase involves a delicate balance requiring synthesis more than lysis. Synthesis is greatly energy dependent, and any depletion of nutrients will push the balance toward lysis and affect the healing process. Excess fibrosis at this stage results in hypertrophic scarring (with the scar limited to the wound area) or keloid formation (with the scar extending beyond wound edge). The difficulty in treating both of these entities has targeted many research dollars on the prevention of scarring, and is discussed by Douglas Sidle, in detail in an article elsewhere in this issue.

Primary and Secondary Healing

It is important to discuss in brief the differences between primary and secondary healing. Primary healing is that which is seen in surgical wounds that involve uncomplicated healing of noninfected, well-approximated wounds (**Fig. 7**). These wounds follow the 4 phases of healing without abruption. Any disruptions in healing such as infection, dehiscence, hypoxia, or immune dysfunction will lead to a compromised wound that enters a stage of secondary healing.[10,11] If no intervention is undertaken, these wounds may become chronic wounds. Chronic wounds are out of the purview

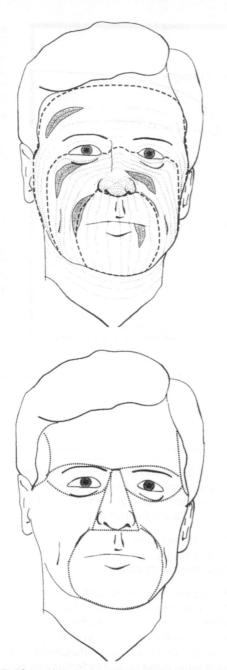

Fig. 7. The relaxed skin tension lines and facial subunit are helpful to plan incisions to achieve optimal appearance of scars. (*Reprinted from* Hom DB, Odland R. Prognosis for facial scarring. In: Harahap M, editor. Surgical techniques for cutaneous scar revision. New York: Marcel Dekker; 2000. p. 31; with permission.)

of this article but they warrant a comprehensive approach for treatment, which obviates the need to monitor surgical wounds. One needs to monitor for the two most common complications, bleeding and infection, using the old tenets of "dolor, rubor,

tumor, and calor" (pain, redness, growth, and heat).[10] Healing by secondary intention, as discussed previously, involves creation of granulation tissue and epithelialization over this healthy granulation tissue. Because angiogenesis and epithelialization takes longer in this setting, they are more prone to infection and poor healing. With proper care, healing by secondary intention may result in acceptable cosmesis on concave surfaces of the face.

Collagen in Wound Healing

Collagen is the single most abundant protein in mammals, and accounts for approximately 30% of our body's total protein content. Collagen and its triple helical structure have been studied for decades, and its structure was first described in the 1930s. Collagen is made from 3 alpha strands of left-handed helices that coil together to form the right-handed helix of a collagen fibril. These fibrils cross-link together via hydrogen bonds to form fibers. The molecular structure of collagen, as for all proteins, is essentially amino acids. The regular arrangement of collagen amino acids (Gly-Pro-X) provides for a great amount of noncovalent bonding. The most important step in the synthesis of collagen is the vitamin C–dependent hydroxylation of the proline. It is this step that provides the tensile strength of collagen and, consequently, wound healing. The depletion of vitamin C in sailors led to scurvy and, ultimately, to poor wound healing and loss of dentition in this population. This major step is also inhibited by systemic steroids, thus resulting in poor wound strength and delayed healing. Hyperbaric oxygen also acts at this step, catalyzing the hydroxylation and improving wound strength as well as accelerating healing.

Wound Strength

Wound strength follows a typical curve in an ideal situation (**Fig. 8**). As one can see, the wound strength begins to plateau around 4 to 5 weeks, reaching around 60% of its original strength. Once healed, it reaches its maximum strength (only 80% of its original) at approximately 1 year.[12] This curve has important implications when selecting suture material to primarily close incisions when material such as Vicryl loses the majority of its strength at 1 month. Sutures are used to close gaping wounds, prevent hemorrhage and infection, support wound strength, and provide an aesthetically pleasing result. The major delineations between materials are monofilament versus multifilament and absorbable versus nonabsorbable. The biomaterial characteristics of different suture material and the time for which

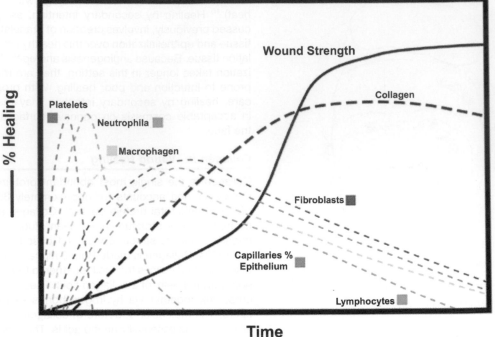

Fig. 8. The typical curve of the increase in wound tensile strength as time progresses. Strength plateaus around 4 to 5 weeks and reaches only 80% of its original strength. (*Reprinted from* emedicine: Wound healing, chronic wounds. Available at: http://emedicine.medscape.com/article/1298452-overview; with permission.)

tensile strength is no longer needed in wound closure is important for choosing the best suture material. One of the basics is the desire to close the wound with suture that will maintain its strength until the wound itself begins to plateau on the tensile curve (4–5 weeks). This time varies—less for mucosal surfaces and more for areas of tension—hence the need for differing suture materials for these areas.

Cytokines in Wound Healing

Cytokines are important signaling molecules that are essential to the healing process. Our current understanding of wound healing has shown the important effects of cytokines; however, most of our knowledge is from in vitro studies. More than 30 cytokines are involved in wound healing produced by macrophages, platelets, fibroblasts, epidermal cells, and neutrophils.[10] Our ability to predict and modify the expression of these cytokines has been much the focus. Future skin scar research is active, especially in the role of transforming growth factor (TGF)-β and the different subtypes that can either impair healing or accelerate healing. The key to the clinical applications of this research will be the cytokine delivery method and the timing of application.

Basic Tenets of Wound Healing

To optimize wound healing there are several basic tenets that one can follow. Winter,[13] in studying epithelialization in pigs, noted 3 critical factors important for the healing of cutaneous wounds:

1. Wound hydration
2. Blood supply
3. Infection minimization.

The ability of ointments and occlusive dressings to trap moisture in the wound has been shown to double the speed of epithelialization.[14] This process prevents desiccation of the upper dermis and allows for more rapid epithelialization. A rolled wound edge is the clinical indicator that epithelialization has been halted. By freshening the wound edge, it helps stimulate and transform the quiescent epithelial cells into migrating keratinocytes to travel over the wound bed. The epithelial layer serves as a physical barrier to prevent infection and desiccation.

Intrinsic and Extrinsic Factors in Wound Healing

Factors affecting wound healing can be divided into intrinsic and extrinsic factors (**Box 1**). Intrinsic

Box 1
A nonexhaustive list of the intrinsic and extrinsic factors that affect healing

Intrinsic factors

- Age
  - Fetus
  - Child
  - Adult
- Immune status
- Hypertrophic scarring and keloids
- Psychophysiological stress
  - Stress
  - Pain
  - Noise
- Hereditary healing diseases
  - Ehlers-Danlos syndrome
  - Epidermolysis bullosa
  - Marfan syndrome
  - Osteogenesis imperfecta
  - Werner syndrome
- Disease states
  - Chronic pulmonary disease
  - Chronic cardiac disease
  - Chronic liver disease (cirrhosis)
  - Uremia
  - Alcoholism
  - Diabetes
  - Peripheral vascular disease

Extrinsic factors

- Malnutrition
  - Protein-calorie
  - Vitamins
  - Minerals
- Infection
- Insufficient oxygenation or perfusion
  - Hypoxemia
  - Hypoxia
  - Anemia
  - Hypovolemia
- Smoking
- Cancer
- Radiation
- Chemotherapy
- Medications
  - Steroids
  - Anticoagulants
  - Penicillamine
  - Cyclosporine

Reprinted from Hom DB, Odland R. Prognosis for facial scarring. In: Harahap M, editor. Surgical techniques for cutaneous scar revision. New York: Marcel Dekker; 2000. p. 25–37; with permission.

factors are those related to the overall health of the patient and any predisposing factors. In general, any connective tissue and inflammatory disorders influence wound healing, such as in any patient with alterations in the key components of wound healing including leukocytes, protein production, and relative or actual immunodeficiencies (human immunodeficiency virus, diabetes, and so forth). Other obvious factors that decrease wound healing are chronic or acute diseased states including liver disease, uremia, malignancy, sepsis, and shock. Patients affected by these conditions may have limited ability to mount an immune response, provide less oxygenation to healing tissues, or have a diminished nutritional supply for the healing process.

AGE IN WOUND HEALING

As we age, our ability to heal decreases as a result of decreased collagen density, fewer fibroblasts, increased elastin fragmentation, and slower wound contraction. Age-related healing was reportedly first studied in World War I by P. Lacompte du Nouy, who noted that it took almost twice as long for a 40-year-old man to close a 40-cm^2 wound than for his 20-year-old compatriot. Although his studies did not involve controls for many variables, it did begin the focus on age-related changes in the skin and their effects on healing.

As we age, the total amount of collagen in the dermis decreases by 1% per year. The epidermal turnover time decreases as well, most dramatically after the age of 50. The dermis also becomes relatively acellular and avascular. These age-related changes, along with the many systemic diseases that occur later in life, all translate into slower and less effective healing.[15]

INFECTION IN WOUND HEALING

Preventing infections in wounds includes debriding necrotic tissue, absorbing exudate, and decreasing bacterial colonization. Bacterial load greater than 10^5 per gram of tissue leads to infection and delayed healing.[16] The goal of wound care is to keep the bacterial load below this critical value, achieved by lightly packing any dead space in the wound and using gentle dressings to most appropriately treat the wound, thus preventing accumulation of any exudates that can be a nidus for infection. Diverting salivary flow is important in preventing exposure of the wound to enzymes and oral flora. The plethora of available wound dressings to prevent infection is out of the purview of this article.

IMMUNE FUNCTION IN WOUND HEALING

Whether alterations to immune function are intrinsic or extrinsic, their effect on the inflammatory phase of healing leads to poor wound healing. Immunosuppressed individuals are less able to fight infection but also lack proper functioning or quantity of inflammatory cells to proper follow the inflammatory phase. If improper cellular debridement of the wound occurs via these cells, wound healing is delayed and ultimately leads to more scarring.

Exogenous use of anti-inflammatory medications can alter the healing environment within the first 3 days of healing. Essential molecular modulators are released within these first 3 days of the inflammatory phase, and any medications that alter this phase will, in turn, alter healing. Corticosteroids, immunosuppressants, or chemotherapy agents are the prime culprits. In practice, it is optimal to have patients off these medications for at least 1 month before surgery and for at least 1 to 2 weeks after surgery. Once the inflammatory phase has concluded, it is less essential to be off these medications.[17]

DIABETES AND WOUND HEALING

Diabetics have poor wound healing for many reasons. Decreased perfusion caused by accelerated atherosclerosis and neuropathy make diabetic patients an increased risk for infection. Along with decreased immune function, this sets up a scenario for prolonged and abnormal healing. Besides the obvious immune dysfunction, diabetics also have slower collagen synthesis and accumulation, decreased angiogenesis, and poorer tensile strength of wounds, leading to higher rate of dehiscence. Tight control of hyperglycemia is essential in the diabetic healing wound, sometimes even necessitating hospitalization and endocrine consultation.

HYPERTROPHIC SCARRING AND KELOIDS

Although keloids are discussed in other articles in this publication (see "Keloids: Prevention and Management" by Sidle and Kim), they deserve mention here for their role in predicting scarring based on patient factors. Hypertrophic scars and keloids are the result of an enhanced proliferative phase of healing and decreased collagen lysis, which are the end result of excessive immature collagen (type III) and especially ECM (water and glycoprotein) deposition. Hypertrophic scars stay within the boundaries of the original wound, whereas keloids extend beyond the limits of the wound. Both entities have been found in all races, but tend to affect darker-pigmented individuals. Of note, keloids have not yet been reported in albinos. African Americans have the highest rate of keloid formation (6%–16%). Although they can occur anywhere, the body areas most susceptible to this abnormal scarring include the earlobe, angle of mandible, upper back and shoulders, upper arms, and anterior chest. Hormonal factors play a role, as they usually are prominent only in women during the fertile years (puberty to menopause). Increased areas of wound tension are also susceptible, thus reiterating the need for tension-free closures. Concern for the development of keloid is in the third week when the proliferative phase appears to continue unabatedly. At this point it is difficult to determine whether keloid or hypertrophic scar will occur and, despite extensive research, it is still undetermined as to what causes the transition from one to the other. TGF-β seems to play a large role in keloid formation, as there is enhanced mRNA expression of TGF-β1 in keloid tissue.[18]

OXYGEN DELIVERY IN WOUND HEALING

Perfusion and oxygenation are the key elements of wound healing and are the two most common reasons for failure of wound healing. Oxygen is key in many steps of the wound-healing process including inflammation, bactericidal activity, angiogenesis, epithelialization, and collagen deposition. Collagenases operate best between oxygen levels of 20 and 200 mm Hg, and human incisions average 30 to 40 mm Hg. Any alterations in the delivery of oxygen, such as vasoconstriction due to hypovolemia, catecholamines, stress, and cold slow the course of wound healing. Wounds of the head and face as well as the anus, compared with extremities, show remarkable healing times because of their high vascularity. Wound Pao_2 can be maximized with increased perfusion and exogenous supplemental oxygen to achieve oxygen levels of 100 mm Hg, which can improve chronic wound healing.[19]

NUTRITION IN WOUND HEALING

Protein and DNA synthesis are essential elements of the healing process. Any diminution of the building blocks (ie, amino acids and nucleic acids) or any cofactors involved in these processes can have detrimental effects on the wound. Malnutrition of any sort can have a strong negative effect but protein deficiency has a profound effect, due to the large amount of collagen synthesis that takes place. A depleted protein status leads to decreased fibroblast proliferation, decreased proteoglycan and collagen synthesis, decreased angiogenesis, and altered collagen remodeling.[6] Albumins of less than 1.5 mg/dL result in poor collagen production and overall poor wound healing.[20] Poor carbohydrate reserve/intake leads to protein catabolism with subsequent depletion of proteins essential to healing. These effects are seen most dramatically in acute malnutrition states (weeks before and after injury). Vitamin deficiencies can also lead to poor healing, especially vitamins C and A, zinc, and thiamine. Vitamin C and thiamine (B1) are essential in collagen formation, and deficiencies lead to decreased cross-linking and, ultimately, wound strength. Vitamin A is essential to the inflammatory process, but its role is not fully understood. Zinc is another cofactor key to wound healing that should be supplemented in the perioperative period, especially in high-risk populations (ie, head and neck cancer). A weight loss of 10% or greater is the general cutoff for severe malnutrition, seen in many of the head and neck cancer patients who require reconstruction. Even a short period of repletive enteral nutrition via nasogastric tube will significantly improve postoperative healing.[21]

SMOKING IN WOUND HEALING

Smoking has long been known to affect the healing process. It is believed that besides the direct toxic effects of the constituents of cigarettes, the most harm results from the generalized vasoconstrictive effects of nicotine. Sorenson and colleagues[22] studied 78 smokers for 15 weeks and divided them into 3 groups. The first group smoked 20 cigarettes a day before and in the weeks following wounding. The next group smoked 20 cigarettes a day before and used a nicotine patch after wounding. The last group was abstinent throughout. The infection rate of the 2 smoking groups was 12% compared with 2% in the nonsmokers. In fact, abstinence for 4 weeks prior to wounding resulted in a dramatic decrease in infection but no change in wound dehiscence. Nonsmokers did not have any wound dehiscence. Smoking has been shown to decrease the function of neutrophils, inhibit collagen synthesis, and increase levels of carboxy-hemoglobin. Interestingly enough, nicotine patch users had no adverse events, which led to the conjecture that other components in cigarette smoke contribute to poor healing. In general, most facial surgeons recommend abstinence from smoking for at least 4 to 6 weeks, if not longer, especially when undertaking elective skin-flap surgery.

RADIATION IN WOUND HEALING

Radiation has multiple effects on wound healing, which can be classified as short-term and long-term effects. Radiation in the short term induces a state of microvascular obliteration and fibrosis, and alters cellular replication.[6] Chronic changes are attributable to the effects on blood vessels, causing narrowing of all vessel sizes and vessel wall degeneration. Optimal timing for surgical procedures in radiation patients should be after the acute injury period but before the chronic phase has taken hold. This period translates to between 3 weeks and 3 months following radiation therapy.[21,23]

CHEMOTHERAPY IN WOUND HEALING

These therapeutic agents are directed at altering cellular replication at multiple levels. The cells most affected are those that undergo rapid turnover. Bone marrow suppression of cells directly involved in the healing process are also affected, which results in fewer monocytes and megakaryocytes, and thus fewer circulating platelets and macrophages. Obvious delays in healing result.

FUTURE RESEARCH IN WOUND HEALING

Much of the recent research in wound healing has been on cytokine and chemokine modulation. Much research has been dedicated to the role of TGF-β and its isomers with their differing effects on healing. TGF-β1 was studied by Zugmaier and colleagues[24] when it was given intraperitoneally to nude mouse models for 10 days; this led to marked fibrosis and scarring. Shah and colleagues[25–27] have studied neutralizing antibodies against profibrotic TGF-β1, with good results, and also studied the role of TGF-β3 and its antifibrotic effects. The critical step in this process is to not only understand the type of cytokines to target but also when to target them to most effectively modulate healing.

REFERENCES

1. Sipos P, Gyory H, Hagymasi K, et al. Special wound healing methods used in Ancient Egypt and the mythological background. World J Surg 2004;28:211–6.
2. Mogensen M, Morsy HA, Thrane L, et al. Morphology and epidermal thickness of normal skin imaged by optical coherence tomography. Dermatology 2008;217(1):14–20.
3. Ha RY, Nojima K, Adams WP Jr, et al. Analysis of facial skin thickness: defining the relative thickness index. Plast Reconstr Surg 2005;115(6):1769–73.
4. Hom DB. Wound healing in relation to scarring. Facial Plast Surg Clin North Am 1998;6:11.
5. Larouche D, Lavoie A, Germain L, et al. Identification of epithelial stem cells in vivo and in vitro using keratin 19 and BrdU. Methods in Molecular Biology. In: Turksen K, editor, Epidermal cells, vol. 289. Clifton (NJ): Humana Press; 2005. p. 383–400.
6. Hom DB, Odland R. Prognosis for facial scarring. In: Harahap M, editor. Surgical techniques for cutaneous scar revision. New York: Marcel Dekker; 2000. p. 25–37.
7. Rodero M, Khosrotehrani K. Skin wound healing modulation by macrophages. Int J Clin Exp Pathol 2010;3(7):643–53.

8. Robson MC. Proliferative scarring. Surg Clin North Am 2003;83:557–69.

9. Pilcher BK, Wang M, Welgus HG, et al. Role of matrix metalloproteinases and their inhibition in cutaneous wound healing and allergic contact hypersensitivity. Ann N Y Acad Sci 1999;878:12–24.

10. Kujath P, Michelsen A. Wounds—from physiology to wound dressing. Dtsch Arztebl Int 2008;105(13): 239–48.

11. Hom DB, Hebda PA, Gosain AK, et al. Essential tissue healing of the face and neck. Shelton (CT): BC Decker and People's Medical Publishing House; 2009.

12. Franz MG, Kuhn MA, Robson MC, et al. Use of the wound healing trajectory as an outcome determinant for acute wound healing. Wound Repair Regen 2000;8(6):511–6.

13. Winter G. Formation of the scab and the rate of epithelialization of superficial wounds in the skin of young domestic pig. Nature 1962;193:293.

14. Alvarez OM, Mertz PM, Eaglstein WH. The effect of occlusive dressings on collagen synthesis and re-epithelialization in superficial wounds. J Surg Res 1983;35(2):142–8.

15. Fenske NA, Lober CW. Structural and functional changes of normal aging skin. J Am Acad Dermatol 1986;15(4):571–85.

16. Robson MC. Wound infection: a failure of wound healing caused by an imbalance of bacteria. Surg Clin North Am 1997;77:637–50.

17. Stadelmann WK, Digenis AG, Tobin GR. Impediments to wound healing. Am J Surg 1998;176(2A Suppl):39S–47S.

18. Abdou AG, Maraee AH, Al-Bara AM, et al. Immunohistochemical Expression of TGF-β1 in Keloids and Hypertrophic Scars. The American Journal of Dermatopathology 2011;33(1):84–91.

19. Schreml S, Szeimies RM, Prantl L, et al. Oxygen in acute and chronic wound healing. Br J Dermatol 2010;163(2):257–68.

20. Otranto M, Souza-Netto I, Aquila MB, et al. Male and female rats with severe protein restriction present delayed wound healing. Appl Physiol Nutr Metab 2009;34(6):1023–31.

21. Payne WG, Naidu DK, Wheeler CK, et al. Wound healing in patients with cancer. Eplasty 2008;8:e9.

22. Sorenson LT, Karlsmark T, Gottrup F. Abstinence from smoking reduces incisional wound infection: a randomized control trial. Ann Surg 2003;238(1): 1–5.

23. Hom DB, Adams GL, Monyak D. Irradiated soft tissue and its management. Otolaryngol Clin North Am 1995;28(5):1003–19.

24. Zugmaier G, Paik S, Wilding G, et al. Transforming growth fact beta-1 induces cachexia and systemic fibrosis without an anti-tumor effect in nude mice. Cancer Res 1991;51:3590–4.

25. Shah M, Foreman D, Ferguson MW. Reduction of scar tissue formation in adult rodent wound healing by manipulation of the growth factor profile. J Cell Biochem 1991;S15F:198.

26. Shah M, Foreman D, Ferguson MW. Control of scarring in adult wounds by neutralizing antibody to transforming growth factor β. Lancet 1992;339: 213–4.

27. Shah M, Foreman D, Ferguson MW. Neutralization of TGFB-1 and TGFB-2 or exogenous edition of TGFB-3 to cutaneous rat wounds reduces scarring. J Cell Sci 1995;108:985.

Scar Revision Techniques: Z-Plasty, W-Plasty, and Geometric Broken Line Closure

William W. Shockley, MD

KEYWORDS

- Facial scars • Scar revision • Z-plasty
- Facial plastic surgery technique

Most scars are traumatic in nature and their length and orientation result from the initial injury and repair. The scar reflects the degree and depth of the injury and whether or not the skin edges were torn, frayed, or beveled. The amount of skin loss affects not only the appearance of the scar but the degree of distortion involving adjacent structures. In addition to the extent of injury and soft-tissue loss, there are multiple other factors affecting the degree of the scar deformity. These factors include the orientation of the scar, the position of the scar with respect to facial landmarks, the age of patient, the genetic factors affecting healing and scar formation, and the techniques used in wound closure.[1]

Scar revision procedures are designed to optimize the appearance of the scar. An ideal scar is one that is thin and flat, has a good color match with the surrounding skin, and is oriented along the relaxed skin tension lines (RSTLs). Scar revision procedures are designed to change the characteristics of the scar in such a way that it becomes a more ideal scar. There are limitations imposed by the shape and size of the scar, neighboring facial landmarks, and the variabilities of healing.

In counseling patients about scar revision, it is important to emphasize that the procedure is designed to trade a poor scar for a better scar. Misconceptions about creating an invisible scar must be corrected.

This article addresses the use of scar revision surgery as it relates to irregularization techniques. Each of these is discussed in detail and the author will provide his perspectives with respect to the indications, advantages, and limitations of each procedure.

TIMING OF SCAR REVISION

Scars tend to improve spontaneously as they mature. The timing of scar revision has traditionally been in the range of 6 to 12 months; however, for some scars there is enough deformity that consideration can be given for earlier scar revision. One rule of thumb is what the author and colleagues have termed the plateau phenomenon; that is, if patients and the physician observe the scar over a 2- to 3-month period and there is no significant improvement, a decision can be made as to whether scar revision is indicated. Typically, scar revision is not performed before 3 months following injury. It is important to note the resolution of the acute inflammatory changes in the tissues surrounding the scar. The adjacent skin should be soft, supple, and nontender. Ideally, there should be no significant residual erythema, edema, or induration.

The necessity and timing of scar revision is a joint decision made by the physician and the patient. The role of the physician is to inform and educate patients about what options exist and

Facial Plastic and Reconstructive Surgery, Department of Otolaryngology/Head and Neck Surgery, University of North Carolina School of Medicine, CB # 7070, G105 Physicians Office Building, 170 Manning Drive, Chapel Hill, NC 27599-7070, USA
E-mail address: william_shockley@med.unc.edu

Facial Plast Surg Clin N Am 19 (2011) 455–463
doi:10.1016/j.fsc.2011.06.002
1064-7406/11/$ – see front matter © 2011 Elsevier Inc. All rights reserved.

what degree of improvement can be expected. If there is a question about whether scar revision is indicated, it is always best to err on the side of waiting. In general, scars improve over time, and unless there are functional issues, there is usually no downside to further observation before surgical intervention is entertained.

TYPES OF SCAR DEFORMITIES

The spectrum of posttraumatic scar deformities is quite significant. Some scars are hypertrophic, being thick, wide, and raised. Atrophic scars are thin, wide, and flat. Scars may be depressed, stellate, or multinodular (lumpy bumpy). On occasion, patients may develop a thin scar, but it might have a poor color match or be oriented in the wrong direction. Scars can also be associated with distortion of adjacent structures, such as misalignment of the vermilion border, traction on the nasal ala, or creating a contour deformity of the lower eyelid. The author's classification system is shown in (**Table 1**).[2]

SCAR REVISION TECHNIQUES

It is important for the surgeon to identify the problematic nature of the scar: whether it is raised, too wide, too thin, depressed, causing distortion of a facial landmark, or running perpendicular to the relaxed skin tension lines. Once the decision has been made to proceed with the scar revision, the goals of the procedure should be identified (**Table 2**).

Multiple surgical procedures have been described to improve facial scars. These procedures include scar repositioning, simple excision, serial excision, and the 3 techniques discussed here. This article

Table 2
Goals of scar revision

Make the scar narrower and flatter
Reorient or reposition the scar
Fill in the depression
Break up the scar
Smooth out an irregular scar
Improve the color of the scar
Correct facial landmark distortion

focuses on irregularization techniques: Z-plasty, W-plasty, and geometric broken line closure (GBLC). The goals of this article are to provide the reader with the indications for each specific technique, the advantages these techniques offer, and the limitations that are inherent with each technique. In addition, practical tips with respect to the planning and execution of each operative technique are discussed.

Z-PLASTY

Z-plasty can be used to help reorient a scar so that the new scar lies in a more favorable position with respect to the relaxed skin tension lines. The Z-plasty procedure represents a double transposition flap, where the scar to be excised lies along the central limb of the Z-plasty with 2 peripheral limbs of equal length placed parallel to each other (**Fig. 1**). The resulting central limb will be perpendicular to the original scar.

Clinical Application

The indications for Z-plasty include scars that are greater than 30° off the RTSLs, scars that are contracted, and scars that form webs. With the classic Z-plasty, each limb is the same length and the angles of the 2 triangular flaps are 60°. Given these parameters, for any given scar there are 2 options for designing the limbs of the Z. It is important to choose the option that will result in the new scars lying in a more favorable position with respect to the RSTLs (**Fig. 2**). On the face, the 3 limbs of the Z are designed to be equal, each being 5 mm in length. The nature of the Z-plasty precludes the entire scar from being parallel to the RSTLs. In addition to improving the orientation of the scar, a multiple Z-plasty breaks up the scar. This irregularization and new orientation makes the scar less conspicuous. Although there is little scientific evidence related to scar revision procedures, it would seem to make sense that creating different vectors of tension might be an advantage in avoiding scar hypertrophy and contraction.

Table 1
Types of scar deformities

Scar	Deformity
Hypertrophic scar	Thick, raised
Atrophic scar	Thin, flat
Depressed scar	Indented
Irregular scar	Multinodular, stellate, and so forth
Poorly oriented scar	Good scar, wrong direction
Scar with poor color match	Good scar, wrong color
Scar associated with distortion of adjacent structure	Elevation of brow, traction on nasal ala, and so forth

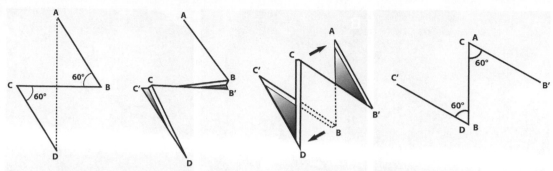

Fig. 1. Classic 60° Z-plasty with equal limbs, before and after transposition of flaps.

Z-plasties can be planned as single or multiple. For a long scar, multiple Z-plasties can be applied in either an interrupted or serial (contiguous) fashion. On the face, it is better to make multiple small Z-plasties than to create fewer Z-plasties with large limbs. When using the multiple Z-plasty as a serial technique, the planned incisions run parallel to the limbs of the Z-plasty at either end of the scar. It should be noted, however, that with the serial Z-plasty technique, the flaps become 3-sided rhombic flaps, not 2-sided triangles (**Fig. 3**). This technique results in flaps that may require trimming and adjustment as they are transposed. Another word of caution is that the limbs of these flaps become longer. The limbs in between the 2 peripheral limbs become approximately twice as long as the limbs before transposition (eg, 5 mm limbs become 10 mm limbs). This concept is illustrated in **Fig. 4**.

In special circumstances, an additional advantage of the Z-plasty technique is that it will provide added length in the axis of the original scar. For this reason, Z-plasties are good for contracted scars as well as webbed scars. As any good resident knows, the angle used for Z-plasty varies directly with the ideal increase in length. For example, using 30° angles will increase the length by 25%, 45° angles are associated with a 50% increase and 60° angles increase the ideal length by 75%. These numbers are based on theoretical and mathematical models. In the clinical setting, the true additional length is less than the theoretical length because of the elasticity of the adjacent tissues.

Advantages

The advantages of Z-plasty include reorientation of the scar, lengthening the scar, and irregularization of longer scars. One additional advantage of Z-plasty over W-plasty or GBLC is that there is minimal to no excision of normal tissue with the Z-plasty, whereas the other 2 techniques require additional skin excision.

Limitations

The disadvantages of a Z-plasty are self-evident. Once the scar is excised and a Z-plasty is created, the scar becomes 3 times as long as the original

Before   **After**

A

B

= original scar   = RSTLs

Fig. 2. Scar to be excised with limbs applied at 60° angles. Two options exist for a Z-plasty (*A, B*). Result following transposition of flaps shows that option (*A*) results in a more favorable orientation.

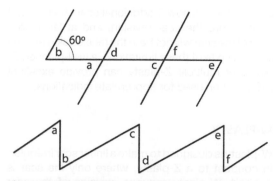

Fig. 3. Serial Z-plasties demonstrating elongation of the limbs as well as transposition of quadrangular flaps.

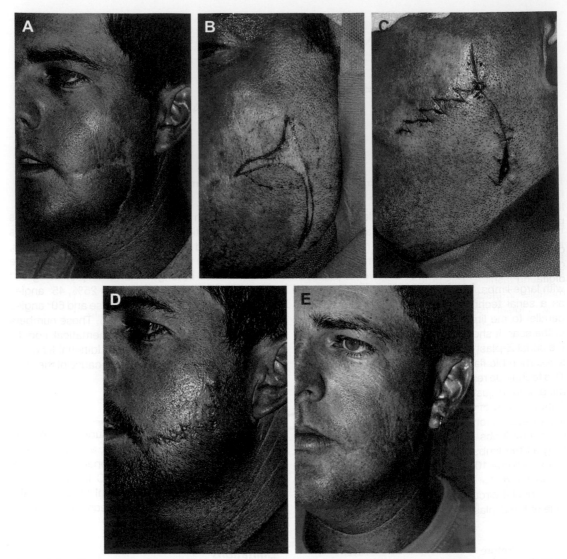

Fig. 4. (*A*) Stellate scar left cheek with significant depression. (*B*) Planned scar excision. Circle denotes soft-tissue depression in the area of planned augmentation. (*C*) Initial closure following insertion of allograft dermis. Serial and multiple Z-plasties were also used. (*D*) Result at 1 week following suture removal. (*E*) Result at 6 months.

scar. There are now 2 additional scars that did not exist before the scar revision, and at least one-third of the scar will not be in the relaxed skin tension lines. In spite of these limitations, a well-planned Z-plasty or multiple Z-plasty can provide excellent results when used for appropriate indications.

W-PLASTY

W-plasty is designed to make a linear scar irregular. In contrast to a Z-plasty, where only the scar is excised, W-plasty requires excision of the scar and additional adjacent normal skin. **Fig. 5** demonstrates the concept of the W-plasty technique.

Clinical Application

The indications for W-plasty include short scars that run against the RSTLs; scars over curved surfaces, such as the inferior border of the mandible; closures in the pretrichial area; and scars or incisions along concave surfaces where webbing and cicatricial healing is predicted.[3] Some investigators feel this technique is also suited for U-shaped scars demonstrating the trap door deformity.[4] The procedure has the most utility when used for scars in areas of skin laxity (eg, forehead, temple, cheeks, and chin).

The W-plasty procedure consists of a series of small triangular advancement flaps on either side

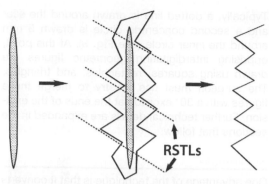

Fig. 5. Excision of scar using W-plasty technique. Some limbs of the W can be planned along RSTLs. Scar, proposed excision, closure with completion of W-plasty.

of the scar. The scar is excised and multiple triangles are created so that closure occurs in an interdigitating fashion. This procedure is different from multiple Z-plasties where the triangular and quadrangular flaps are transposed. W-plasty is an advancement flap, whereas a Z-plasty is a transposition flap. The limbs of the W-plasty can be planned in such a way that many of them fall into the RSTLs (see **Fig. 5**). It is important that the W-plasty is created in such a way that there is a 30° angle at each end to avoid a dog ear.

One additional qualification is that the W-plasty should only be done in areas of the face where there is sufficient laxity to allow the bilateral advancement flaps. Typically, this would be the cheek, forehead, chin, and temple (**Fig. 6**). It is important to emphasize that additional soft tissue is excised at the time of scar revision; thus, clinical judgment will dictate whether this additional skin excision will be associated with excessive wound tension at the time of skin closure.

Advantages

Advantages of the W-plasty are that it is easy to plan and construct and it is straightforward regarding its execution. The primary advantage is that it can break up a linear scar into smaller segments, many of which run parallel to the RSTLs. One technical challenge comes in creating the ends of the W-plasty. As mentioned, it is important to have the scar excision tapering to 30° angles at each end. There may be occasions where it is advantageous to use a fusiform excision that is perpendicular to the distal end of the W-plasty. This excision will obviate having to use 30° excisions. One investigator also described diminishing the length of the W-plasty limbs toward the ends of

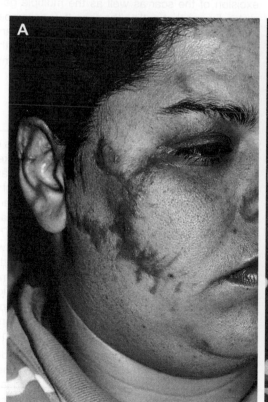

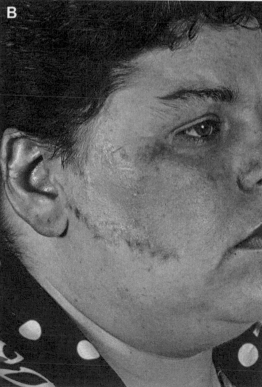

Fig. 6. (*A*) Extensive traumatic scars right cheek with widening and hypertrophic changes. (*B*) Postoperative result at 12 months following W-plasty revision of multiple scars, performed in 2 stages to minimize wound tension.

the excised skin (**Fig. 7**), thus, creating a more fusiform defect, facilitating closure without a standing cutaneous deformity.[3]

Limitations

The disadvantage of the running W-plasty is that it creates a scar that has a regular repetitive pattern and, therefore, may be more noticeable. For this reason, the W-plasty technique works well for shorter scars, but it is not as well suited for long facial scars.

GEOMETRIC BROKEN LINE CLOSURE

This procedure is designed to excise the scar and create a randomly irregular scar. This technique is particularly indicated for long scars that lie in a poor orientation with respect to the relaxed skin tension lines.

Clinical Application

The scar is excised using interdigitating geometric lines, drawn in such a fashion that triangles, rectangles, and squares are created in a random pattern (**Fig. 8**). Creating a pattern where some of the lines follow the RSTLs further optimizes the ultimate scar. Bilateral advancement flaps are created with undermining of the soft tissues, and the design itself facilitates closure with interdigitation of the geometric figures. Although some investigators incorporate semicircles, this author typically uses only angulated figures. As with the W-plasty, each end must include a *v* that is less than 30°. This procedure obviates the dog-ear that will likely occur if a wider angle is used. Creating significant angulation with random irregularity, the scar is less noticeable than the scars resulting from other scar revision techniques, including the multiple Z-plasty and running W-plasty.

The indications for GBLC include long scars that are poorly oriented with respect to the RSTLs. It is generally accepted that the scar should be greater than 30° off of the RSTLs. Because additional excision of normal tissue is required, the GBLC technique should only be considered in areas where there is sufficient skin redundancy and elasticity for closure without tension.

Cupp and colleagues[5] provided a detailed description for the design of the GBLC technique.

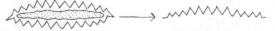

Fig. 7. W-plasty technique with limbs of diminishing size allowing for a more fusiform excision, thus minimizing problems with a standing cutaneous deformity at either end.

Typically, a dotted line is drawn around the scar and a second concentric circle is drawn 5 mm around the inner circle (see **Fig. 8**). At this point, opposing interdigitating geometric figures are drawn using squares, rectangles, and triangles. The surgeon must use artistry to merge these figures with a 30° excision at the ends of the excision. Further technical details are expanded in the sections that follow.

Advantages

One advantage of the technique is that it converts a long, easily visible scar into a scar broken up into multiple short segments (**Fig. 9**). Some of the new scar now lies in a more favorable position. However, the primary advantage is that the new scar is randomly irregular, making the scar less noticeable because the eye has more difficulty tracking this irregular, multiply segmented line.

Limitations

The disadvantages of the GBLC technique are twofold. It is the most complex approach regarding planning, designing, and executing the procedure. In addition, by its nature the technique is only useful when there is sufficient adjacent skin to allow for excision of the scar as well as the multiple geometric figures that outline the scar. If, for example, the scar was 2 mm wide and the rectangles and triangles were 4 to 5 mm from the edge of the scar, then the skin excision would be 10 to 12 mm in width.

PRINCIPLES OF SCAR REVISION
Preoperative Planning

As with any procedure, preoperative planning is of critical importance. Photographs should be taken and the deformity carefully analyzed. There are several reconstructive options, and after thoughtful planning, the surgeon should consider each of these and choose the one most appropriate for the particular scar and its orientation. The proposed scar revision technique should be drawn out on the patients' photograph along with the RSTLs. At this time, one can anticipate problems, such as tension vectors, dog-ears, and distortion of adjacent structures. If any significant problems are identified at this phase, alternate or additional procedures can be planned before any incisions are made.

Preparation Prior to Incision

This author performs the surgical preparation first, followed by marking the scar and the proposed excision. Important facial landmarks are identified

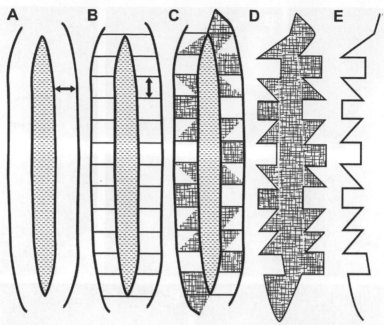

Fig. 8. (*A*) Scar with lines drawn 5 mm beyond either side of scar. (*B*) Horizontal lines drawn 5 mm apart. (*C*) Proposed excision of scar with geometric design. (*D*) Defect following excision of scar as well as 360° undermining. (*E*) Resulting geometric broken line following closure. (*Adapted from* Cupp CL, Johnson MB, Larrabee WF, et al. Scar revision. Facial Plast Surg Clin North Am 1998;6(2):195–201; with permission [*D*].)

and, if necessary, are marked before the injection of local anesthesia because this often distorts subtle landmarks, such as the vermilion border. The scar revision plan is carefully marked out using a fine-tip marking pen. It is important to infiltrate the lidocaine with epinephrine solution into the mid dermis to create vasoconstriction and to enhance tissue turgor, which aids in making fine cuts with the scalpel. It is also important to inject in such a way that the marked area is not affected, so that the fine lines remain intact. The RSTLs are identified and can also be marked. It is important during the injection process to avoid smudging the preoperative markings.

Incisions and Closure

Depending on the scar revision technique used, either a #15 or #11 blade can be used. The initial incision is made just into the upper dermis until the entire circumference has been incised. This procedure allows for sufficient tension for the incision to be made. With W-plasties and GBLCs, one can incise from the apex at the point of the figure into the scar itself (from inside to outside). The scar and adjacent tissues are then excised at the subdermal level, leaving behind a scar platform that will prevent problems with depression of the new scar. At this point, the tissues are undermined

in a 360° fashion, typically using a scalpel, undermining the immediate subdermal plane. A small guarded bipolar is used to attain hemostasis. With scar irregularization techniques, such as Z-plasty, W-plasty and GBLC, the tips of the flap are sutured to the appropriate corners. Deep sutures are placed as deemed appropriate. The remaining defect is closed with running 6-0 locking or simple interrupted sutures.

Posttreatment Care

In the immediate postoperative period, patients may clean the incision with hydrogen peroxide and then apply topical antibiotic ointment. The author's personal preference for those patients undergoing irregularization scar revision is to apply Mastisol (Ferndale Laboratories, Ferndale, MI, USA) and Steri-strips (3M Healthcare, St Paul, MN, USA) along the axis of the scar. This practice serves as an occlusive dressing and eliminates the need for patients to perform wound care. It seems to allow the small flaps to be compressed in a uniform fashion because there is often some subtle irregularity with respect to the levels of the flaps. The Steri-strips are removed 5 to 7 days later, and any permanent sutures are removed.

The patients undergoing scar revision should avoid the sun for at least 6 months, which means

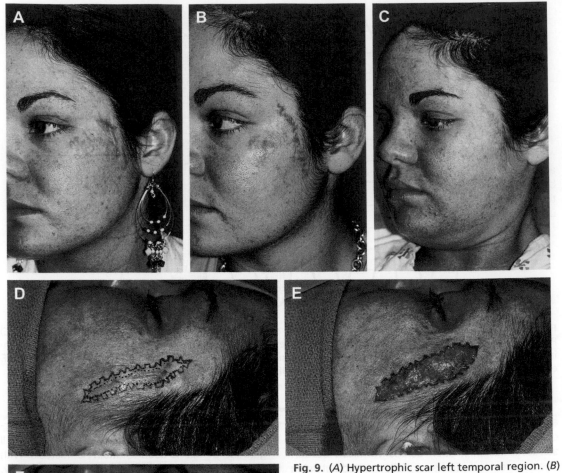

Fig. 9. (*A*) Hypertrophic scar left temporal region. (*B*) Initial result at 2 months. (*C*) Result at 6 months. (*D*) Proposed geometric design for excision of scar. (*E*) Immediate result following excision of scar. Note expansion of defect. (*F*) Result following undermining and closure.

avoiding direct sun exposure as well as the liberal use of sunscreens. Scar massage may enhance the ultimate result by improving the mobility of the soft tissues and helping to minimize lymphedema. Numerous topical treatments also exist for minimizing scar deformity. These treatments include silicone gels, topical steroid creams, topical steroid tape, vitamin E preparations, and Mederma (Merz Pharmaceuticals, Greensboro, NC, USA).

Mederma has been promoted in direct consumer advertising but its evidence-based efficacy is still a matter of debate. The reader is encouraged to read the contributions in this journal by Drs Tristani and Patel for further perspectives on the use of this topical therapy.

Not uncommonly, adjunctive procedures may follow this type of scar revision surgery. The most common techniques are dermabrasion and laser resurfacing. These techniques are typically performed 8 weeks following scar revision. This author prefers dermabrasion because of its simplicity, safety, and low cost. Following scar revision, dermabrasion helps to smudge the scar borders and flatten the hills and valleys of the scar.

Z-plasty, W-plasty, and Geometric Broken Line Closure

Three types of scar irregularization techniques are considered. Each of these has its own indications, advantages, and limitations. The surgeon should be experienced with each of these and preoperatively decide which, if any, is appropriate for a particular scar in a given patient. As with any technique, careful preoperative planning along with meticulous execution will lead to optimal results.

REFERENCES

1. Kokoska MS, Thomas JR. Scar revision. In: Papel ID, editor. Facial plastic and reconstructive surgery. 3rd edition. New York: Thieme; 2009. p. 59–65.
2. Shockley WW. Scar revision techniques. Operative Techniques in Otolaryngology-Head and Neck Surgery 2011;22(1):84–93.
3. Park SS. Scar revision through W-plasty. Facial Plast Surg Clin North Am 1998;6(2):157–61.
4. Borges AF. W-plasty. Ann Plast Surg 1979;3(2):153–9.
5. Cupp CL, Johnson MB, Larrabee WF, et al. Scar revision. Facial Plast Surg Clin North Am 1998;6(2):195–201.

Elegant Solutions for Complex Paramedian Forehead Flap Reconstruction

Nathan Todd Nelson Schreiber, MD,
Steven Ross Mobley, MD*

KEYWORDS

- Paramedian forehead flap • Nasal reconstruction • Alar rim
- Cartilage graft • Surgical delay • Topical nitroglycerin
- Steroid injection • Nasal scars

Elegant solutions are frequently sought by both artists and engineers. In dance, for example, elegance is defined by the minimum amount of motion that results in the maximum visual effect. Similarly, engineers strive to provide simple and practical solutions to their challenges while efficiently balancing the demands of time, materials, and other constraints. The confluence of art and engineering is never more intertwined than it is in complex multistage nasal reconstruction. The surgeon must draw on both the practical and scientific qualities of an engineer and the creativity of an artist. Experienced surgeons can quickly identify challenges, craft efficient solutions, and optimize reconstructive benefits for their patients with each surgery. In short, experienced surgeons reconstruct complex nasal defects with the most elegant of solutions.

The basic principles and techniques of facial reconstruction have been in use and relatively unchanged for a surprising number of years. As early as the fourth century, a Byzantine physician named Oribasius described advancement flaps, recognized the importance of tension-free closure, and warned of complications in poor wound healers, the elderly, and individuals in generally poor health.[1] Because the human eye can perceive asymmetries of only millimeters, the modern facial plastic surgeon must be creative and precise to recreate facial symmetry as much as is humanly possible.

In evaluating a patient for facial reconstructive surgery, the reconstructive ladder of increasing complexity and surgical involvement must always be discussed and patients must be guided to the surgical option that best suits their needs and goals. A skin defect can be closed primarily, allowed to heal by secondary intention, repaired with a split or full-thickness skin graft, or reconstructed with a local, regional, or free flap. This article describes refinements in the technique of paramedian forehead flap (PMFF) nasal reconstruction by the senior author (SRM) over his years of practice in a university setting.

PREOPERATIVE PLANNING

There are several factors to consider before initiating any discussion of reconstructive options for a specific patient. In patients undergoing Mohs surgery, the margins should be pathologically clear before reconstruction. If there is a significant risk of recurrence, methods of reconstruction may be suggested that allow for easy monitoring, such as skin grafting. In such a case, a more cosmetically

The authors have nothing to disclose.
Division of Otolaryngology–Head and Neck Surgery, University of Utah Health Sciences Center, 50 North Medical Drive, School of Medicine 3C120, Salt Lake City, UT 84132, USA
* Corresponding author.
E-mail address: steven.mobley@hsc.utah.edu

Facial Plast Surg Clin N Am 19 (2011) 465–479
doi:10.1016/j.fsc.2011.06.003

acceptable definitive reconstruction can be deferred to a later date.

Certain patient populations have poor peripheral circulation, putting them at risk for flap necrosis. Risk factors that cause endothelial dysfunction and impaired neoangiogenesis include tobacco use, poorly controlled diabetes, and irradiation.[2,3] Tobacco use, in particular, increases the risk of flap necrosis and skin slough, and this has been well documented in patients who have undergone rhytidectomy.[4,5] A study in patients undergoing breast reconstruction with a transverse rectus abdominis muscle flap suggests the results are best when a patient abstains from smoking for at least 4 weeks both preoperatively and postoperatively.[6] We also advise our patients to abstain from smoking for a minimum of 4 weeks both preoperatively and postoperatively. However, because many Mohs reconstructions present with little forewarning, the smoking status of the patient must be factored into a safe reconstructive plan, with the performance of a delayed PMFF often the method of choice in a patient who smokes.

THE DELAY PHENOMENON

The practice of surgical delay improving a flap's viability has long been noted. Surgical delay seems to cause several mostly transient effects, including division of sympathetic nerves causing initial release and then depletion of adrenergic factors from nerve endings, vasodilation occurring parallel to the long axis of the flap, ischemic conditioning, blunted release of vasoconstrictive metabolites, and, later, neoangiogenesis. Animal studies have reported maximally increased blood flow at the distal ends of random pattern flaps in as few as 4 days and lasting as long as 14 days.[7–11] Most relevant human studies have investigated breast reconstruction and generally endorse best results with a delay of 7 to 14 days.[12,13] We currently recommend a delay of 7 to 10 days and have a low threshold to perform a delay stage before reconstruction for at-risk patients. It is often difficult for both the surgeon and the patient to commit to surgical delay because of the additional stage of reconstruction that is required. However, we strongly believe that the addition of a delay stage before a given reconstruction can significantly decrease the chances of a flap-related complication. As otolaryngologists, many of us were taught, "If you think of a tracheotomy, perform a tracheotomy"; as facial plastic surgeons, we offer the perspective, "If you think of a delay stage, perform a delay stage." The

additional cost of a delay stage is worth the prevention of distal flap necrosis and the multiple surgeries often required for its repair.

SURGICAL TECHNIQUE
General Principles

It is important to think of the face in terms of aesthetic subunits and to approach each reconstruction with these in mind. As much as possible, incisions should be placed at the borders of aesthetic subunits where they are least noticeable. Generally, a scar within a subunit is more obvious than a scar located at a border between subunits. As a result, the best reconstruction may involve removing additional tissue and rebuilding an entire subunit if the defect involves 50% or more of that subunit.[14] However, there are some exceptions, and a blind adherence to the 50% rule should be no substitute for an artistic reconstructive eye. For example, with lighter skin color, such as Fitzpatrick type I or II, a scar may be placed across a subunit without being noticed as much as with darker skin color. In addition, in contrast to thinner nasal skin, thicker sebaceous nasal skin can be a poor match with the forehead. In this situation, a PMFF might not be the best choice for reconstruction, and one may wish to avoid excising the remaining portion of a subunit if it would make the difference in requiring a pedicled flap for coverage.[15]

PMFF

The PMFF is extremely useful for nasal defects with a diameter larger than 1.5 cm because it can provide a significant amount of nasal coverage with minimal donor defect and is usually an ideal color match for the nose. The flap is centered on the supratrochlear vessels at the medial canthus and should be about 1.2 cm in width at its base. A foil template should be created to match the defect and outlined at the forehead with adequate length to reach the defect in a tension-free manner. The flap can then be elevated and inset. The pedicle can be safely divided and inset 3 weeks later. For full-thickness defects that involve the intranasal lining, the PMFF can be folded over to close the intranasal defect as an alternative to full-thickness skin grafting or a mucosal flap.[16–18] In this situation, a 3-stage operation can be performed at 3-week intervals with delayed placement of a large auricular cartilage batten graft in stage 2. A large cartilage graft, preferably from the septum, abutting the nasal sidewall is often used to provide extra support and prevent collapse.

Surgical Instrumentation

In our experience, the 6900 Beaver blade (Becton, Dickinson and Company (C), Waltham, MA, USA) is a very useful instrument for soft tissue reconstruction of the face and has several applications in PMFF surgery. Unlike the more common 11 and 15 blades, the 6900 Beaver blade is not as widely used. Surgeons who may not be familiar with this particular blade are encouraged to experiment with its use. In soft tissue work, the surgeon can stab into the tissue similar to using an 11 blade. The 6900 Beaver blade, however, is narrower and allows for the creation of precisely sized pockets for the cartilage grafts often used in PMFF nasal reconstruction. In addition, the 6900 Beaver blade is similar in feel to the 15C blade with the added advantage of being able to cut in all directions. Because the 6900 Beaver blade cuts on all sides, it does not need to be continually reinserted when creating a cartilage graft pocket, thereby promoting operative efficiency. The qualities of this blade allow the surgeon to hold it much like a pencil or paintbrush and paint through the soft tissue with artistic precision, cutting with both forward and backward strokes as well as delicate

stabbing advancements. We have found this blade particularly helpful in creating tight pockets to receive the alar rim grafts commonly used in PMFF surgery (**Fig. 1**).

The 6900 Beaver blade is also an excellent instrument for thinning flaps, which is important for achieving a well-contoured final result. The senior author (SRM) originally thinned flaps after their elevation from the forehead using sharp serrated scissors.[19–22] However, we have found it more efficient to thin the PMFF as it is initially raised from the forehead. In this situation, as the flap is being raised off the frontalis musculature, there is extra tension along the flap that, combined with the 6900 Beaver blade, provides an excellent opportunity for flap thinning as it is initially raised. In this technique, the perimeter of the flap is created with either 11 or 15C blade scalpels. Small double-pronged skin hooks are then placed along the edge of the flap for upward tension while the surgeon sits at the head of the bed with the patient's forehead positioned such that both the surface and the immediate underside of the flap can easily be viewed with a simple shift of the surgeon's gaze. In this manner, the 6900 Beaver

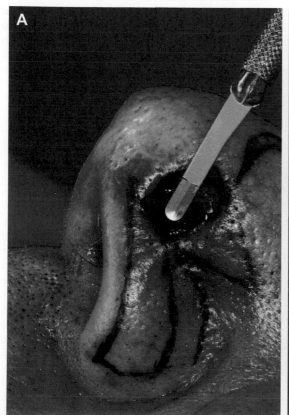 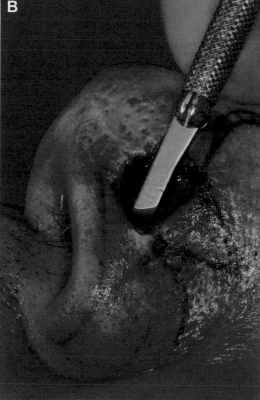

Fig. 1. The 6900 Beaver blade is able to cut on all sides (*A*) and can be used to create a pocket for an alar rim cartilage graft (*B*).

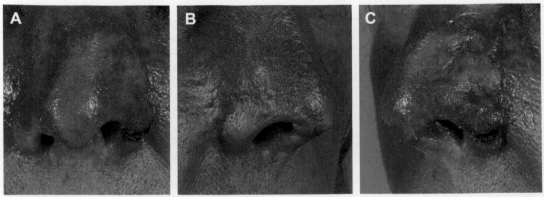

Fig. 2. Asymmetry from distal necrosis of PMFF reconstruction of the left alar rim is shown in frontal (*A*), right three-quarter (*B*) and left three-quarter (*C*) profile views.

blade is gently stabbed into the tissue, leaving 1 to 3 mm of subcutaneous fat on the underside of the forehead flap. The surgeon can watch from below as the blade precisely enters the subcutaneous fat layer and then watch the skin surface of the flap as the blade causes the skin to gently rise, similar to what is seen when the tips of a face-lift scissor press on the underside of the cheek skin during wide undermining. The ability to paint this blade back and forth while gently advancing has allowed us to safely and more quickly raise nicely thinned flaps. These thinner flaps eventually result in a superior contour match. Another advantage of

this technique is that subcutaneous fat and fronta-lis muscle are left in place at the patient's fore-head, which can more quickly provide a healthy base of living tissue on which granulation tissue can more quickly form when the forehead defect cannot be closed primarily and must heal by secondary intention.

Achieving Alar Rim Symmetry, Skin Layer

In PMFF reconstruction of the alar subunit, alar retraction is a significant complication that the facial plastic surgeon must work diligently to

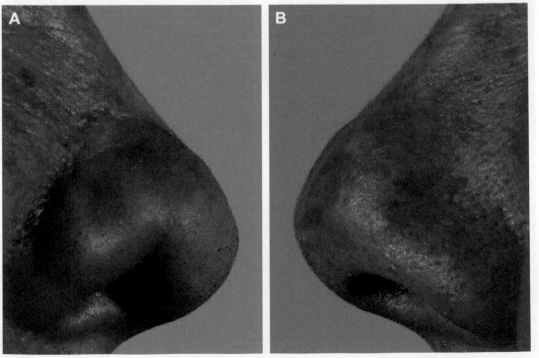

Fig. 3. Retraction after PMFF reconstruction of the right alar rim resulting in a notched right alar rim (*A*) compared to the native left alar rim (*B*).

prevent. In one published study, alar retraction was reported to occur as often as 40% of the time after alar rim reconstruction.[23] Even subtle alar retraction can significantly reduce the elegance of the final surgical result.

Achieving symmetric alar rims is made all the more difficult when a full-thickness defect that involves the alar rim must be repaired. The classic teaching for PMFF nasal subunit reconstruction has been to create a flap that exactly replaces the tissue and/or subunit that has been removed. Through a busy PMFF reconstruction practice dealing with many full-thickness defects, the senior author (SRM) prefers to use a folded PMFF for most of his full-thickness alar subunit reconstructions and has learned that it is often advantageous to leave an additional 2 to 3 mm of tissue at what will eventually be the alar rim. Leaving this tissue is particularly important when reconstructing the ala of someone with a very high aesthetic standard. The reasoning for this is that during the course of a multistage full-thickness alar subunit reconstruction, the distal part of the flap, which will be the new alar rim, is the part of the flap most vulnerable to distal ischemia and poor wound healing. If classic design of the skin paddle is followed and an exact amount of replacement skin is brought from the forehead to the missing alar subunit, the symmetry of the final reconstruction will be in serious jeopardy if there is any distal flap necrosis resulting in a paucity of tissue at the alar rim (**Figs. 2** and **3**). It is extremely difficult to add an additional 2 to 3 mm of tissue once it has been lost, and the patient can expect multiple additional operations in an effort to reconstruct the missing tissue at the alar rim.

A more elegant solution, however, is to purposefully leave 2 to 3 mm of tissue in the skin paddle in the area of the paddle that will eventually be the alar rim. One can always debulk the alar rim to create near-perfect symmetry, but it is another matter altogether to build it up if there is tissue loss and the rim retracts.

Achieving Alar Rim Symmetry, Cartilage Layer

As the sixteenth century French physician Francois Rabelais once said, "Nature abhors a vacuum." There are many situations in facial reconstruction for which this tenet rings true and perhaps none quite as much as when attempting to reconstruct an alar rim. The nasal ala is actually devoid of cartilage in its lateral inferior region (**Fig. 4**). When a partial or full-thickness defect is present in this area, it is important to reconstruct the area with generously sized alar rim grafts. More importantly, when these grafts are inset along the lateral nasal

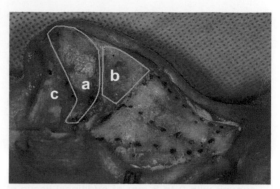

Fig. 4. Nasal dissection in a cadaver showing left lower lateral cartilage (a), upper lateral cartilage (b), and inferior lateral region of nasal ala that normally does not contain any cartilage (c).

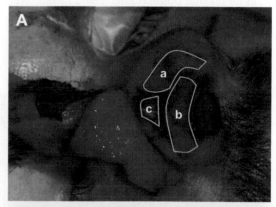

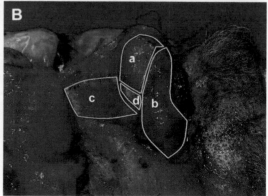

Fig. 5. Examples of abutting cartilages in PMFF nasal sidewall and alar rim reconstruction. (*A*) Native right lower lateral cartilage (a); right alar rim reconstruction with generous auricular cartilage graft, filling the area normally composed of fibrofatty tissue (b); and right upper lateral cartilage reconstruction with septal cartilage graft (c). (*B*) Right lower lateral cartilage reconstruction with auricular cartilage graft (a), right alar rim reconstruction with auricular cartilage graft (b), right upper lateral cartilage reconstruction with septal cartilage graft (c), and septal cartilage graft to eliminate dead space between cartilage grafts (d). Note how the grafts abut one another with little to no gaps.

sidewall, it is imperative that there are no soft tissue gaps between abutting edges of cartilage grafts (**Fig. 5**). If gaps are left between adjacent cartilage grafts, the sidewall can contract, obliterating the dead space and leaving behind a retracted nasal ala.

In patients with high aesthetic standards and full-thickness defects involving the alar rim, repair is planned as follows (**Fig. 6**):

1. Design folded PMFF using a template to reconstruct missing internal lining as well as alar subunit with 2 to 3 mm of additional tissue at what will be the alar rim.
2. If the patient is a smoker or otherwise perceived to be at risk for flap failure, there should be a delay stage, and the PMFF should be sutured in its original position after being raised. Wait 7 to 10 days for the next stage.
3. Raise the folded PMFF to the nose to reconstruct the internal lining and alar subunit. Reconstruct

such that 2 to 3 mm of additional tissue is located at the alar rim. Wait 3 weeks for the next stage.
4. Divide the internal lining from the external skin paddle, and place delayed primary cartilage grafts to support the alar rim, nasal sidewall, tip, and so forth. Wait an additional 3 weeks for the next stage.
5. Divide the pedicle, and inset the flap. Wait 2 months for the final stage.
6. Design a symmetric alar rim and remove any excessive tissue to match the native side (**Fig. 7**).

Supra-Alar Crease

Through-and-through quilting sutures are an important technique for the control of contour that is necessary for complex nasal reconstruction. These through-and-through sutures can have an important and significant effect on the final nasal contour in key areas such as the supra-alar crease. Although the quilting sutures are able to apply

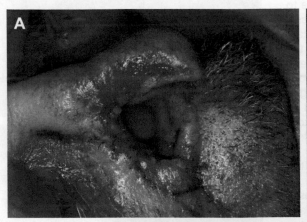
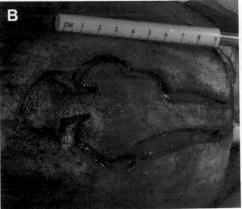
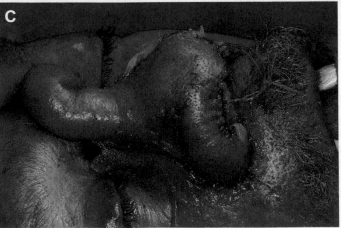

Fig. 6. Folded PMFF nasal reconstruction stage 1. Full-thickness nasal defect (*A*) and planned folded PMFF (*B*) followed by completed reconstruction (*C*) after placement of cartilage grafts and creation of supra-alar crease with quilting sutures (before use of polytetrafluoroethylene pledgets) are shown.

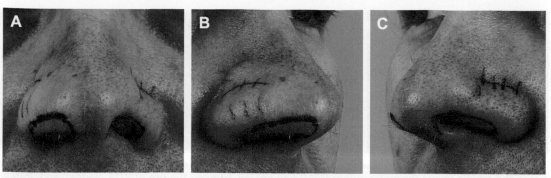

Fig. 7. Result of right alar rim reconstruction with PMFF before final debulking. Markings show planned location of final alar rim in the frontal (A) and right three-quarter (B) profile views. The left three-quarter profile view is shown for comparison (C).

pressure in a precise location, these sutures can have a cheese wire cutting effect on the skin. Alternatively, cotton bolsters have been advocated for this use to help apply broader pressure in the postoperative period without the cheese wire effect.[22] The senior author's (SRM) long-time surgical assistant, Brent Klev, RN, helped suggest an even more elegant solution to control nasal contour. This simple modification combines the benefits of applying pressure in a precise location while at the same time avoiding the cheese wire effect.

In this modification, a 5-0 black nylon is threaded over a polytetrafluoroethylene (PTFE) pledget that is used to precisely place pressure. This not only provides equal, if not superior, soft tissue compression compared with simple quilting but also prevents cheese wiring that occurs when stitches alone are used to create this crease (**Fig. 8**). In addition, the PTFE pledget has 2 ready-made perforations through which the needle can easily be passed such that equal pressure can be placed over the entire area of the pledget. PTFE pledgets

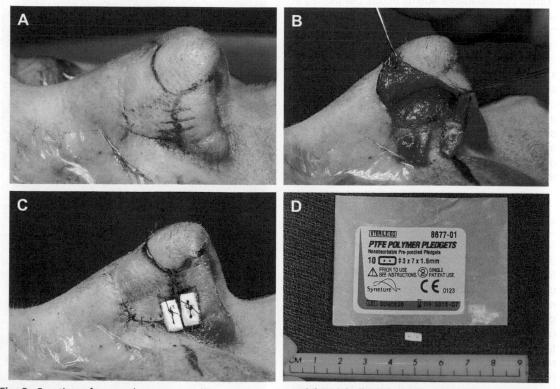

Fig. 8. Creation of supra-alar crease. Bulky supra-alar tissue (A) is debulked through planned incisions (B), and PTFE pledgets are placed to maintain pressure at the planned supra-alar crease (C). The dimensions of the PTFE pledget are shown (D).

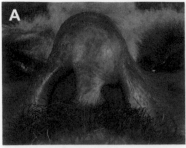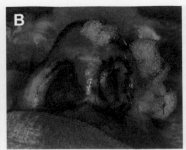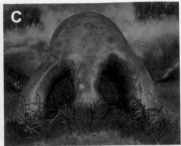

Fig. 9. Preoperative (*A*), intraoperative (*B*), and postoperative (*C*) images of nasal vestibular stenosis repair. Note that in the middle image the senior author (SRM) had not yet adopted the use of PTFE pledget, and, instead, a bulky sponge was used. (*Modified from* Daines SM, Hamilton GS, Mobley SR. A graded approach to repairing the stenotic nasal vestibule. Arch Facial Plastic Surg 2010;12:336. Copyright © 2010 American Medical Association. All rights reserved; with permission.)

are specifically designed to prevent the suture from tearing through the tissue and are used most often in cardiothoracic and vascular surgeries. As a result, otolaryngologists and facial plastic surgeons may not have been widely exposed to the utility of PTFE pledgets in the operating room. PTFE pledgets are best used for this purpose by tying them such that they are just held in place with just the smallest amount of initial tissue compression. That way, in the days after surgery, the compression becomes more appropriate as normal postoperative edema enters the tissues in the days after the flap surgery. A short learning curve can be anticipated by surgeons learning to use PTFE pledgets for soft tissue contour compression. We routinely leave these pledgets in for 5 to 8 days postoperatively and have not seen postoperative complications from excessive compression or cheese wire cutting of tissue. In a minority of cases, the sutures may tighten, causing the pledgets to excessively depress the skin with postoperative edema. If this situation occurs, the pledgets may be removed sooner than the 5 to 8 days they are normally left in place.

Nasal Vestibular Stenosis

Nasal vestibular stenosis can occur to varying degrees after full-thickness repair of nasal ala defects with folded PMFFs and is best prevented by using large autologous grafts in the area of the nasal sidewall and ala. However, despite a surgeon's best efforts, this complication may still occur. Nasal vestibular stenosis in the setting of trauma can be difficult to repair, has a high rate of recurrence, and can often result in significant functional impairment.[24] The senior author (SRM) has had success repairing nasal vestibular stenosis using a batten graft to support the inherently weak nasal ala and a thermoplastic splint for 2

weeks (**Fig. 9**).[25] Alar vestibular stenosis caused by burns and other trauma are less common but can be corrected using the same technique.

POSTOPERATIVE CARE
Topical Nitroglycerin

Flap necrosis is a difficult complication that can significantly delay final repair and lead to

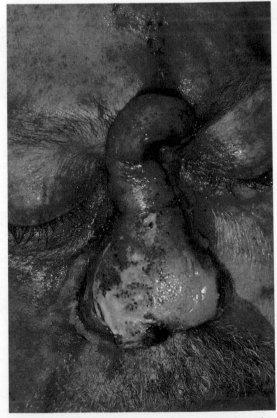

Fig. 10. Topical nitroglycerin used on the distal portion of a PMFF.

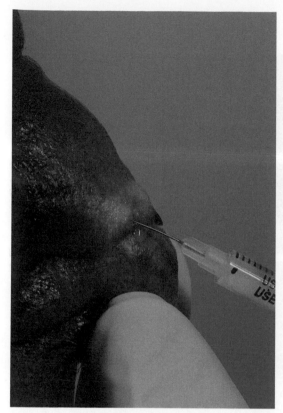

Fig. 11. Injection of triamcinolone to treat pincushion edema of a nasal flap.

radicals that cause both arterial and venous vaso-dilation (**Fig. 10**). Topical nitroglycerin has shown efficacy in improved skin flap survival in several animal models.[26–29] Importantly, a single postoperative treatment with topical nitroglycerin showed no benefit over placebo in flap necrosis for Mohs reconstruction in the only published clinical study to date.[30] Our patients are instructed to use topical nitroglycerin every 4 to 6 hours if their flaps show signs of inadequate perfusion postoperatively. Patients are asked to continue this application for 4 to 6 days or until a more stable flap color is observed. The senior author (SRM) has used this technique for several years in a variety of patients with a spectrum of comorbidities without any significant cardiovascular complications. Patients are instructed to apply a pea-sized amount of paste, about 1 mm thick, over the pale or congested flap and must be warned that most people experience an annoying but tolerable headache. Anecdotally, this method seems to work slightly better for arterial insufficiency as opposed to venous congestion.

Triamcinolone

Pincushioning is often the result of edema and inadequate flap thinning and can reduce reconstruction camouflage. Triamcinolone injections that are intradermal or immediately subdermal can help reduce pincushioning through the useful side effects of lipolysis and inhibition of lipogenesis. Before these injections, however, the patient must be informed of possible complications, such as telangiectasias, hypopigmentation, and skin breakdown.[31] These complications tend to occur

a prolonged course caring for an open wound. One technique that has been useful for the senior author (SRM) is the use of nitroglycerin paste, which is absorbed topically, creating nitric oxide

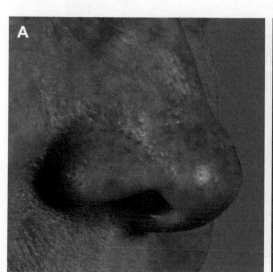

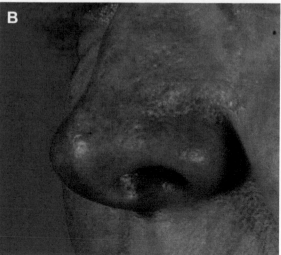

Fig. 12. Opposing three-quarter views allow comparison of nasal ala. A small amount of alar retraction can be seen at the reconstructed right alar rim (*A*) compared to the left (*B*).

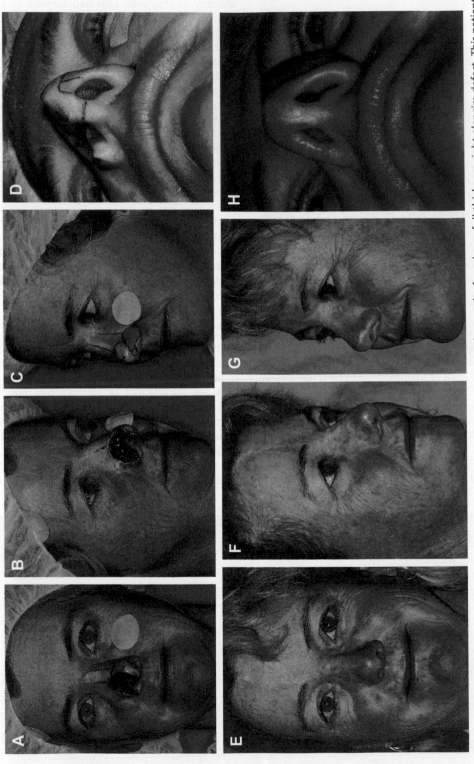

Fig. 13. Comparison of preoperative (A–D) and 4-year postoperative (E–H) PMFF reconstruction results for a large full-thickness right alar rim defect. This patient developed alar retraction with a notched appearance similar to that in **Fig. 3**, requiring additional reconstructive procedures.

with higher concentrations of triamcinolone, such as 40 mg/mL. Telangiectasias may appear a month or more after injection and can even enlarge for up to 6 months.[32] Hypopigmentation related to steroid injection appears in multiple case reports, mainly in the orthopedic literature in which steroid doses are significantly higher than those used by the senior author (SRM).[33] This effect is caused by decreased melanocyte function and is usually temporary and rarely permanent.[34] Nevertheless, hypopigmentation can be particularly disconcerting and especially noticeable in darker-skinned individuals. The risk of skin breakdown, which is especially high in patients with thin skin, is reduced by starting with low concentrations of triamcinolone. With the concentrations we use, we have seen a few cases of telangiectasias and a little hypopigmentation but no skin breakdown.

We usually begin with triamcinolone at a final concentration of 2.5 mg/mL (mixed with lidocaine and bicarbonate for patient comfort) in 0.1-mL aliquot injections from a 1-mL tuberculin-type syringe for each approximate 5 mm² of edema. The first injection is administered at 3 to 6 weeks

postoperatively to the deep dermis or top layer of subcutaneous fat. When injected intradermally, the surgeon should see skin blanching (**Fig. 11**). The patient is followed up for 4 weeks, and, if no appreciable effect is noticed, an increased triamcinolone concentration of 5 mg/mL can be injected, continuing with 0.1-mL aliquots per each approximate 5 mm² of persistent tissue edema. There is a definite art to this technique, and the learning surgeon is advised to proceed slowly, spreading treatments over longer intervals, perhaps 6 weeks initially, until comfort is gained with how much edema resolves with a given injection. The possibility of injecting more triamcinolone at a later time is a particularly important concept with this technique.

REPORTING RESULTS
Photography

It would be difficult to overstate the importance of photography in facial plastic surgery. Standardized and consistent photographs allow each surgeon to more accurately assess and report their forehead

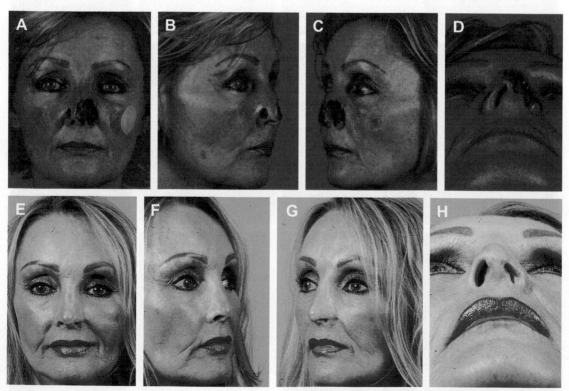

Fig. 14. Comparison of preoperative (*A–D*) and 5-year postoperative (*E–H*) reconstruction results for a superficial right alar defect repaired with a melolabial flap and a large full-thickness left alar rim defect repaired with a PMFF. This patient's reconstruction was complicated by distal necrosis of the PMFF, shown in **Fig. 2**, requiring additional reconstructive procedures.

flap reconstruction results to the professional community at large. Ideally, photographs are taken of a patient without makeup or expression; after removing jewelry, hats, and other accessories; and at well-defined angles.[35] In addition, nonadherence to standard practices in photography can lead to the publication of possibly misleading results. For example, variations of only 10° from standard camera angles can shorten or lengthen various facial features to a significant degree, resulting in distorted assessment.[36] Nasal skin cancer reconstruction photos, and especially those involving the alar rim, can fall victim to publication of nonstandardized photography results. To

ensure the most accurate assessment of a given postoperative result, the contralateral ala should always be shown juxtaposed to the reconstructed ala. Without showing the unaffected side, subtle amounts of alar rim retraction, which are quite noticeable on direct observation, can be blinded to the observer of the published photo. We encourage all nasal reconstruction results involving repair on or near the ala to be published or presented with the contralateral ala opposite to the reconstructed result (**Fig. 12**). The adoption of this standard will ensure that the results of given reconstructive techniques are more objectively presented.

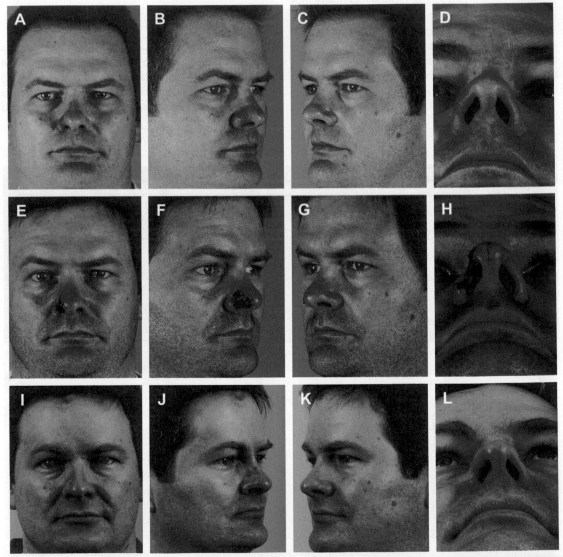

Fig. 15. Comparison of preresection (*A–D*), postresection/preoperative (*E–H*) and 1-year postoperative (*I–L*) PMFF reconstruction results for a full-thickness right alar rim defect. Appearance after reconstruction but before final debulking is shown in **Fig. 7.**

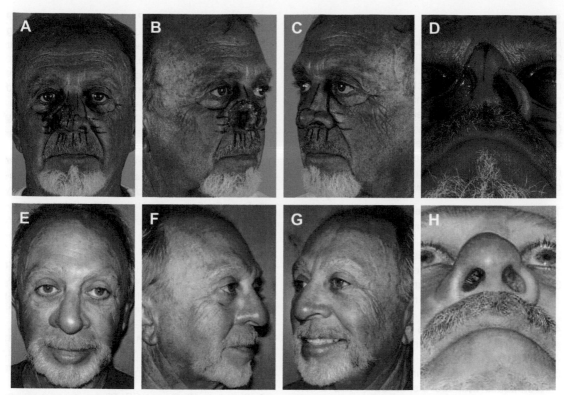

Fig. 16. Comparison of preoperative (*A–D*) and 7-month postoperative (*E–H*) PMFF reconstruction results for a large full-thickness right alar rim defect. Note that only preoperative images with surgical markings and postoperative images taken by the patient at home due to a long travel distance and inability to followup in clinic were available. Intraoperative reconstruction images are shown in **Fig. 6**.

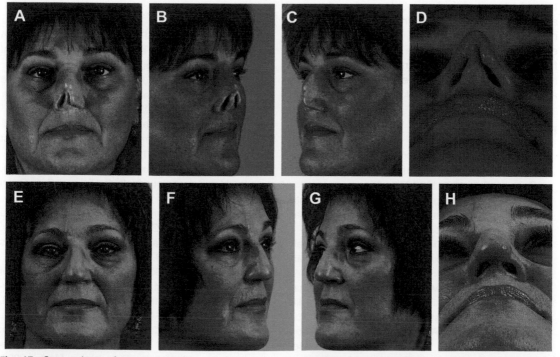

Fig. 17. Comparison of preoperative (*A–D*) and 10-month postoperative (*E–H*) PMFF reconstruction results for a long-standing, bilateral, full-thickness alar rim and nasal tip defect.

SUMMARY

Reconstruction of nasal defects is a particularly challenging task, requiring the reconstructive surgeon to recreate facial symmetry to within millimeters to reduce detection. The techniques mentioned in this article have been refined over several years and have helped the senior author (SRM) to achieve increasingly symmetric reconstructive results while preventing complications and the need for unplanned surgeries along the reconstructive journey (**Figs. 13–17**). A summary of key principles is as follows:

1. Always provide choices, and help patients choose the reconstructive option that best fits their situation.
2. Consider comorbidities and have a low threshold to add a staged surgical delay.
3. Aim to reconstruct entire subunits, but use an artistic eye and do not adhere to this rule blindly.
4. Add an additional 2 to 3 mm of skin paddle when reconstructing through-and-through defects of the ala.
5. Experiment with the surgical instruments and techniques that are discussed in this article (the 6900 Beaver blade, PTFE pledgets, nitroglycerin paste, and triamcinolone injection) to enhance results.

By following these principles, we have been able to navigate our patients through a series of reconstructive stages that maximizes final aesthetic results while minimizing complications. We encourage the use of these techniques amongst facial plastic surgeons to improve reconstructive results in complex multistage nasal reconstruction and create more elegant solutions for patients.

REFERENCES

1. Lascaratos J, Cohen M, Voros D. Plastic surgery of the face in Byzantium in the fourth century. Plast Reconstr Surg 1998;102:1274–80.
2. Argacha JF, Adamopoulos D, Ghjic M, et al. Acute effects of passive smoking on peripheral vascular function. Hypertension 2008;51:1506–11.
3. Goessler UR, Bugert P, Kassner S, et al. In vitro analysis of radiation-induced dermal wounds. Otolaryngol Head Neck Surg 2010;142:845–50.
4. Rees TD, Liverett DM, Guy CL. The effect of cigarette smoking on skin-flap survival in the face lift patient. Plast Reconstr Surg 1984;73:911–5.
5. Riefkohl R, Wolfe JA, Cox EB, et al. Association between cutaneous occlusive vascular disease, cigarette smoking, and skin slough after rhytidectomy. Plast Reconstr Surg 1986;77:592–5.
6. Chang DW, Reece GP, Wang B, et al. Effect of smoking on complications in patients undergoing free TRAM flap breast reconstruction. Plast Reconstr Surg 2000;105:2374–80.
7. Milton S. The effects of delay on the survival of experimental studies on pedicled skin flaps. Br J Plast Surg 1965;22:244–52.
8. Myers MB, Cherry G. Differences in the delay phenomenon in the rabbit, rat, and pig. Plast Reconstr Surg 1971;47:73–8.
9. Finseth F, Cutting C. An experimental neurovascular island skin flap for the study of the delay phenomenon. Plast Reconstr Surg 1978;61:412–20.
10. Pang CY, Forrest CR, Neligan PC, et al. Augmentation of blood flow in delayed random skin flaps in the pig: effect of length of delay period and angiogenesis. Plast Reconstr Surg 1986;78:68–74.
11. Holzbach T, Neshkova I, Vlaskou D, et al. Searching for the right timing of surgical delay: angiogenesis, vascular endothelial growth factor and perfusion changes in a skin-flap model. J Plast Reconstr Aesthet Surg 2009;62:1534–42.
12. Erdmann D, Sundin BM, Moquin KJ, et al. Delay in unipedicled TRAM flap reconstruction of the breast: a review of 76 consecutive cases. Plast Reconstr Surg 2002;110:762–7.
13. Christiano JG, Rosson GD. Clinical experience with the delay phenomenon in autologous breast reconstruction with the deep inferior epigastric artery perforator flap. Microsurgery 2010;30:526–31.
14. Burget GC, Menick FJ. The subunit principle in nasal reconstruction. Plast Reconstr Surg 1985;76:239–47.
15. Singh DJ, Bartlett SP. Aesthetic considerations in nasal reconstruction and the role of modified nasal subunits. Plast Reconstr Surg 2003;111:639–48.
16. Burget GC, Menick FJ. Nasal support and lining: the marriage of beauty and blood supply. Plast Reconstr Surg 1989;84:189–202.
17. Menick FJ. A 10-year experience in nasal reconstruction with the three-stage forehead flap. Plast Reconstr Surg 2002;109:1839–55.
18. Menick FJ. A new modified method for nasal lining: the Menick technique for folded lining. J Surg Oncol 2006;94:509–14.
19. Burget GC, Menick FJ. Aesthetic reconstruction of the nose. In: Burget GC, Menick FJ, editors. Aesthetics, visual perception, and surgical judgement. St Louis (MO): Mosby; 1993. p. 48.
20. Burget GC, Menick FJ. Aesthetic reconstruction of the nose. In: Burget GC, Menick FJ, editors. The paramedian forehead flap. St Louis (MO): Mosby; 1993. p. 77–9.
21. Baker SR. Local flaps in facial reconstruction. In: Baker SR, editor. Interpolated paramedian forehead flaps. 2nd edition. Philadelphia: Mosby; 2007. p. 284–5, 293–5.

22. Baker SR. Local flaps in facial reconstruction. In: Baker SR, editor. Reconstruction of the nose. 2nd edition. Philadelphia: Mosby; 2007. p. 449–50, 452, 473.

23. Mureau MA, Moolenburgh SE, Levendag PC, et al. Aesthetic and functional outcome following nasal reconstruction. Plast Reconstr Surg 2007;120: 1217–27.

24. Mavili E, Akyurek M. Use of upper lip flap for correction of nostril stenosis. Otolaryngol Head Neck Surg 1999;121:840–1.

25. Daines SM, Hamilton GS, Mobley SR. A graded approach to repairing the stenotic nasal vestibule. Arch Facial Plast Surg 2010;12:332–8.

26. Rohrich RJ, Cherry GW, Spira M. Enhancement of skin-flap survival using nitroglycerine ointment. Plast Reconstr Surg 1984;76:943–8.

27. Nichter LS, Sobieski BA, Edgerton MT. Efficacy of topical nitroglycerine for random-pattern skin-flap salvage. Plast Reconstr Surg 1985;75:847–52.

28. Davis RE, Wachholz JH, Jassir D, et al. Comparison of topical anti-ischemic agents in the salvage of failing random-pattern skin flaps in rats. Arch Facial Plast Surg 1999;1:27–32.

29. Price MA, Pearl RM. Multiagent pharmacotherapy to enhance skin flap survival: lack of additive effect of nitroglycerin and allopurinol. Ann Plast Surg 1994; 33:52–6.

30. Dunn CL, Brodland DG, Griego RD, et al. A single postoperative application of nitroglycerin ointment does not increase survival of cutaneous flaps and grafts. Dermatol Surg 2000;26:425–7.

31. Louis DS, Hankin FM, Eckenrode JF. Cutaneous atrophy after corticosteroid injection. Am Fam Physician 1986;33:183–6.

32. Jarratt MT, Spark RF, Arndt KA. The effects of intradermal steroids on the pituitary-adrenal axis and the skin. J Invest Derm 1974;62:463–6.

33. Okere K, Jones MC. A case of skin hypopigmentation secondary to a corticosteroid injection. South Med J 2006;99:1393–4.

34. Venkatesan P, Fangman WL. Linear hypopigmentation and cutaneous atrophy following intra-articular steroid injections for de Quervain's tendonitis. J Drugs Dermatol 2009;8:492–3.

35. Henderson JL, Larrabee WF Jr, Krieger BD. Photographic standards for facial plastic surgery. Arch Facial Plast Surg 2005;7:331–3.

36. Riml S, Piontke A, Larcher L, et al. Quantification of faults resulting from disregard of standardised facial photography. J Plast Reconstr Aesthet Surg 2011;64(7):898–901.

Use of Makeup, Hairstyles, Glasses, and Prosthetics as Adjuncts to Scar Camouflage

Douglas M. Sidle, MD[a],*, Jennifer R. Decker, MD[b]

KEYWORDS

- Nonoperative • Scar camouflage • Camouflage cosmetics
- Facial prosthetics • Scars • Surgery adjuncts

Key Points

- Although surgery inevitably produces a scar, patients have increasingly high expectations for minimally visible scarring.
- Good wound care including prevention of infection, moisturization, and minimal wound strain are critical to optimal scar formation.
- Petrolatum ointment remains the safest and most commonly used topical treatment during scar healing.
- Silicone has been shown to be effective in minimizing hypertrophic scars and is more effective as sheeting than as a gel.
- Vitamin A ointment may improve scars and reduce pruritis. Vitamin E ointment does not significantly improve scars and may be discouraged owing to sensitivity reactions.
- Other topical treatments, including Mederma, have not been shown to significantly improve scar appearance in clinical trials.
- Pressure dressings reduce hypertrophic scarring in burn wounds. Scar massage may improve pruritis and patient mood but has minimal effect on appearance.
- Camouflaging cosmetics come in a wide range of types for patient-specific uses, including minimizing discoloration and irregularities and creating an overall smooth facial appearance.
- Peripheral scarring may be adequately camouflaged by hairstyling, glasses, or facial hair.
- Facial prosthetics should be considered for craniomaxillofacial defects when surgical reconstruction is not the best option or needs to be delayed.
- Preoperative consultation with a craniomaxillofacial prosthetics center and trained anaplastologists assists in both surgical resection planning and facial prosthetics development.

The authors have no conflicts of interest or financial obligations to disclose.
[a] Division of Facial Plastic Surgery, Department of Otolaryngology–Head and Neck Surgery, Northwestern University Feinberg School of Medicine, Northwestern Memorial Hospital, Chicago, IL, USA
[b] Department of Otolaryngology–Head and Neck Surgery, Northwestern University Feinberg School of Medicine, McGaw Medical Center, Chicago, IL, USA
* Corresponding author. Department of Otolaryngology–Head and Neck Surgery, Northwestern University Feinberg School of Medicine, 676 North St Clair, Suite 1325, Chicago, IL 60611.
E-mail address: drsidle@yahoo.com

Facial Plast Surg Clin N Am 19 (2011) 481–489
doi:10.1016/j.fsc.2011.06.004
1064-7406/11/$ – see front matter

The process of scar formation occurs as an important part of the healing process after damage to the skin's dermal layer, whether through infection, trauma, or surgery. Although scars are both important and inevitable after injury, patients may find them functionally and cosmetically disruptive. Facial scars, in particular, are viewed as undesirable and potentially disfiguring. Research into the psychological effects of facial scarring has shown feelings of decreased self-worth, social self-consciousness, and isolation that persist after wound healing is complete.[1] Distress over the persistence of facial scarring has been shown to have significant long-term quality of life impacts. However, patients also report lack of empathy from the medical community regarding scarring and poor long-term support services.[2]

Facial plastic surgeons are frequently called upon to assist in the management of facial scarring. Although many techniques are present to minimize existing scars, none can erase a scar completely. Thorough explanation of inevitable scar development during consent for any surgical procedure is critical for patient understanding and satisfaction. With proper planning, minimization of scar development and camouflage of its appearance afterward can lead to satisfactory cosmetic outcomes without need for revision. In addition, both patients and physicians need to be aware of the many options available to them to reduce a scar's appearance even after healing is complete.

This article reviews options for nonsurgical treatment of existing scars that can be used by the patient to improve a scar's appearance. Treatments during the healing and maturation processes include occlusive dressings, topical treatments, and massage. Interventions for existing scar camouflage include topical cosmetics, use of hairstyling and glasses, and facial prosthetics. Descriptions of surgical planning and revision techniques, dermabrasion, laser resurfacing, and steroid injections are addressed in other articles (See the articles by William W. Shockley; Surowitz and Shockley; Foo and Tristani-Firouzi; Sobanko and Alster elsewhere in this issue for further exploration of this topic).

HISTORY OF SCAR CAMOUFLAGE

A smooth flawless facial appearance is a primary determinant of health, youth, and beauty in many societies. For centuries, facial powders have been used to lighten and even the skin tone. However, powders do not hide scars well and require frequent reapplications. In seventeenth century Europe, beauty patches were used to cover and distract from disfiguring small pox scars. Facial foundation was later developed primarily for use in the theater to provide long-lasting skin coverage. The first true facial foundation was termed as wet white and incorporated white powder into a thin liquid base foundation. Grease paints were also developed to incorporate color and filler into an oil base for longer wear and coverage.[3]

However, cosmetics continued to be the domain of the theater rather than the general public until Max Factor invented cake makeup in 1936. This compressed powder provided excellent coverage of skin irregularities with a lighter feel and more natural look than grease paints. In addition, the cake was carried in a convenient compact and easily applied with a damp sponge. Suddenly, facial foundation became convenient for the general public.

Since this time, the scope and application of modern facial foundations available has expanded dramatically. As a result, many patients now expect a flawless complexion and any scars to be minimally visible. However, no amount of surgical skill or scar revision can completely eliminate a scar. As a result, foundations have been improved for medical use, tattooing has expanded to include scar coverage, and medical teams have been developed for development of complex facial prosthetics. The modern facial plastic surgeon needs a working knowledge of the techniques available so that patients can make clear informed decisions on how to best camouflage their scar.

TOPICAL SCAR TREATMENT

Scar healing requires several months before the final appearance is created. Early healing involves high levels of fibroblastic activity, which cause deposition of collagen. Erythema may present in the early stages from inflammation or neovascularization. Scars then mature over a period of several months, with the ideal scar being thin, level to surrounding skin, of good color match, and located along subunits or relaxed skin tension lines. Unfavorable scar formation results in noticeable color change, a depressed or raised scar, hypertrophy or keloid formation, or scar widening. Although some scar formation properties are genetic, knowledge of basic healing principles can reduce scar visibility. The surgeon is well aware of the importance of scar planning and meticulous closure techniques to eliminate tension and create skin eversion. However, postoperative care can affect scar formation while involving the patient in the healing process.

Wound Care

Control of concomitant medical issues and prevention of infection can aid in wound healing.[4]

Diabetic patients should closely monitor blood glucose levels. Patients who smoke should be counseled on the likelihood of more difficult healing and to reduce or quit smoking before surgery. Perioperative antibiotics are typically given to prevent infection, which greatly disrupts wound healing and is a predisposing factor for hypertrophic or keloid scars.[5] Wounds should be kept clean with gentle removal of crusting and dirt using cotton swabs and peroxide. As necessary, the wound should be covered to prevent contamination or external trauma.

Dressings

In addition to keeping wounds clean, dressings can improve scar formation. Tape strips may reduce scar widening by preventing micromotion even in the mimetic facial muscles. Early consistent application of moisture through ointments or occlusive dressings aids in cell turnover and epidermal migration over the wound surface.[6] Petroleum ointment is inexpensive and can be applied liberally without the risks of allergic reactions associated with antibiotic ointments.

Silicone

Silicone is the most rigorously studied topical scar improvement agent. In particular, silicone sheeting applied to wounds has been shown to improve wound healing and hypertrophic scar appearance. The silicone sheeting is thought to combine consistent pressure on the wound with an occlusive dressing that increases moisture in the stratum corneum.[7] Doppler study of blood flow in scars with sheeting applied also indicates increased temperature that may assist in perfusion, although measurable blood flow changes are not seen.[8] Silicone sheeting may be worn for 12 to 24 hours per day and may be rinsed and reapplied for up to 2 weeks. In addition, silicone applied as a topical gel has been shown to improve scars during the early healing phase by providing consistent moisture.[9] Although not as effective on hypertrophic scar as sheeting, silicone gel has better patient compliance on visible areas such as the face.[10]

Other Topicals

After initial wound healing and suture removal, patients may wish to apply a range of over-the-counter topical emollients. The most commonly available ointments include antioxidants such as retinoids (vitamin A) or tocols (vitamin E). Topical retinoic acid has been shown to both subjectively and objectively improve hypertrophic and keloid scar appearance.[11] Vitamin E ointments, although commonly used by patients and even encouraged by some physicians, have not been shown to improve scar appearance.[12] In another study, scar appearance worsened and local allergic reactions were noted, leading to discouragement of its use.[13] Herbal extracts containing onions (Allium cepa) and madecassol (Centella asiatica) are also being aggressively marketed; studies have not demonstrated efficacy, but side effects are uncommon.[3] One of the most marketed topical scar treatments Mederma (Merz Pharmaceuticals, Greensboro, NC, USA) is a gel-based onion extract that did not show significant improvement in scar healing or appearance in a randomized double-blinded split-scar study when compared with petroleum ointment.[14]

Massage

Mechanical forces alone can have an effect on scar formation during the remodeling phase. Direct pressure has been shown to reduce inflammation and normalize hypertrophic scar composition and is used frequently in management of burn scars.[15] Massage therapy has a long anecdotal history in management of hypertrophic scars. Most research has been performed in burn patients, in whom massage has been shown to improve pruritis, overall scar status, and patient depression levels.[16] However, a prospective trial in pediatric burn patients with hypertrophic scarring failed to show a significant benefit of massage plus pressure dressing over pressure dressings alone on scar pliability and banding.[17]

CAMOUFLAGING MAKEUP

A wide range of cosmetic products is available and effective for corrective camouflage of facial scars. Cosmetics use 2 principles to conceal a scar: using color theory to diminish a scar or foundation for complete concealment. Although both principles may be used in conjunction, color theory focuses specifically on the scarred area, whereas a foundation must be blended over the entire face.

Color Theory

Every cosmetic choice begins with a base color as close to the patient's natural skin tone as possible. Next, any color abnormalities of the scar area are evaluated, and an undercover cosmetic is applied. Based on the color wheel, the opposite color family should be applied to conceal pigmentary changes: green for an erythematous base, yellow for darkened or ecchymotic areas, or violet for sallow areas of collagen degeneration. As scars have no adnexal structures to assist with adhesion, the cosmetic should be dabbed and pressed firmly into the scar rather than rubbed because this will remove color.[18] After the base foundation is blended, shading and highlighting principles can be used to minimize contour abnormalities. Depressed scars appear darker, so a light powder should be applied. In contrast, hypertrophic scars catch the light and should have a darker powder applied on the most raised areas (**Fig. 1**).

Foundations

Foundations are used over the entire face to blend irregular skin patterns or a large scar. The type of foundation selected is based on the desired characteristics and need for coverage. **Table 1** reviews foundation formulations as well as advantages and disadvantages.[19,20] Surgical cosmetics are those developed for complete opaque coverage for large scars with pigmentary disorders. The most commonly used surgical foundation in the United States is Dermablend (L'Oreal International, Clichy Cedex, France), which is available at many department stores. Surgical foundations tend to be thicker and more occlusive. They have long wear times and can even be used while swimming. In addition, surgical foundations require the application of a specific powder for proper setting and long wear. However, full-face application of any of the more occlusive foundations can result in masklike faces. Central rouge over the nose and cheeks as well as lip and eye color are important to create a sense of depth and a more natural final appearance.

How I do it: camouflage cosmetic application instructions for office use

- Prepare the skin by washing with a gentle cleanser, then create a balanced surface by applying a moisturizer to dry areas and using an astringent for oily areas.
- Apply surgical or tinted foundation to scar areas first using color opposites for tinting. Use color opposites for best camouflage: green to cover erythema, violet to cover sallow skin, yellow to cover darkening or ecchymosis.
- For heavy surgical foundation, apply a small amount to the back of the hand to warm it, then use a fingertip to firmly dab the scar pressing firmly to set the foundation. Allow to dry for 5 minutes before other makeup application.

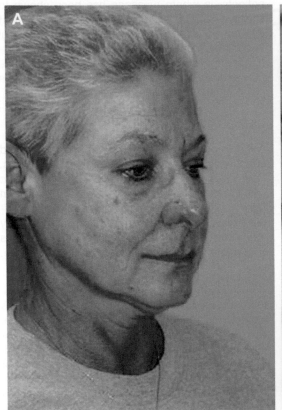
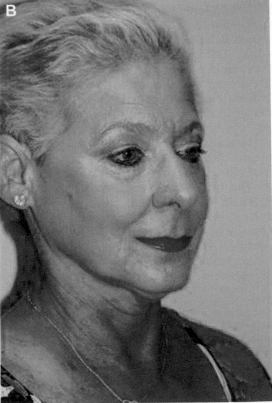

Fig. 1. Right melolabial flap resulted in well-healed but reddened scarring (*A*) that becomes minimally noticeable after green-based scar cover-up followed by foundation (*B*). (*Courtesy of* Dr Douglas Sidle and Northwestern Department of Otolaryngology, Northwestern University, Feinberg School of Medicine, Chicago, IL; with permission.)

Table 1
Cosmetic foundation types

Foundation	Formulation	Advantages	Disadvantages
Water based	Oil emulsified in a water base	• Light feel • Popular for all-day all-over use • Easy to remove	• May change color with wear • Not waterproof
Oil based	Water emulsified in an oil base	• Water resistant • Long wearing, no color change, & moisturizes dry skin	• Moderately greasy • Moderately occlusive • May exacerbate acne
Oil free	Silicone oil emulsified in water (no mineral or vegetable oils)	• Nongreasy feel • Best in acne-prone or oily-skinned patients	• Not waterproof • Mild irritation in some patients
Oil only (anhydrous)	Oils	• Waterproof • Long wearing • Used during swimming & bathing	• Heavy, occlusive • Promotes comedones • Spot coverage best

- Remove a small amount of base foundation. Swipe onto the forehead, cheekbones, nose, and chin.
- Blend to hairline, ears, and beneath the jawline using fingertips. Dab without rubbing over the smooth scar tissue for texture and to set foundation over smooth scar tissue.
- Apply setting powder particularly over scar areas or if using a surgical foundation to prolong adhesion.
- When not needed, cosmetics should be thoroughly removed daily to prevent breakouts.
- Use an oil-based cleanser to fully remove all makeup at nighttime followed by a gentle cleanser and moisturizer.

HAIRSTYLING

Unlike facial skin, forehead and scalp wounds are difficult to manage without obvious scar because of thick dermis and relatively immobile adjacent tissue. In addition, the residual scarring is typically on the facial periphery, outside the central gaze foci of eyes, nose, and mouth, which are more attracted to central scarring or asymmetry.[21] In fact, many heal very well with secondary intention or skin grafting in comparison with large rotational flaps (**Fig. 2**). When managing these wounds, it is important to remember the efficacy of hair in distracting from or covering postoperative scarring. Women typically have more hair, allowing for coverage of many scars in the periphery of face, scalp, and posterior neck as well as near the hairline. Men tend to be able to cover scars in the postauricular area, scalp, and hairline, as well as fine scars in the upper lip (moustache) and lower one-third face (beard). Particularly with forehead wounds, secondary intention healing or skin grafting a combination of hairstyling and cosmetic camouflage techniques can result in satisfactory results using simple surgical means.

GLASSES

The eyes are one of the main sites of gaze, so periocular scars or asymmetries can be perceptible. However, patients who wear glasses may notice significant distraction from the scar simply by their regular use because glasses provide another focus for gaze. Scars most affected by the use of glasses include those on the upper lid, blepharoplasty scars, and paramedian flap or nasal bridge scars. In addition, glasses can cover postauricular scarring from postauricular approaches, facelifts, or parotid surgery.

FACIAL PROSTHETICS

Large facial defects can require significant multistage surgical reconstruction, which may not always be the best choice for the patient. One alternative is facial prosthetic rehabilitation. When considering prosthetics as a temporary or permanent reconstructive option, it is best to refer the patient early to a craniofacial rehabilitation center with experience in designing prosthetics based on individual needs and expectations. Preoperative consultation can assist in recreating the patient's preresection appearance. In addition, coordination between the surgeon and an anaplastologist can optimize surgical resection and

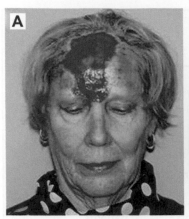
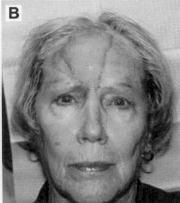
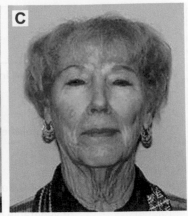

Fig. 2. Large central forehead lesion closed by a split-thickness skin graft and secondary intention (*A*) healed with minimal distortion but visible graft site (*B*). Hairstyling provides significant camouflage (*C*). (*Courtesy of* Dr Douglas Sidle and Northwestern Department of Otolaryngology, Northwestern University, Feinberg School of Medicine, Chicago, IL; with permission.)

closure planning to facilitate prosthetic design, function, and appearance.

Patient Demographics

Many types of patients should be considered for prosthetics as either a temporary or permanent reconstruction option. Patients with poor-quality tissues or significant medical problems may not be good surgical candidates. Other patients prefer the convenience of a prosthesis to multiple staged surgeries (**Fig. 3**). Children may benefit from a prosthesis until they reach an age in which they can participate in the reconstruction decision-making

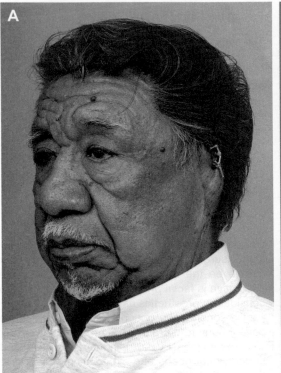
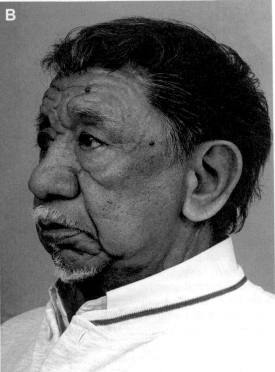

Fig. 3. An adult patient after total auriculectomy (*A*) decided on an ear prosthesis over staged surgical reconstruction, with good cosmetic result (*B*). (Prosthesis fabricated by anaplastologist Rosemary Seelaus.) (*Courtesy of* The Craniofacial Center, University of Illinois at Chicago, Chicago, IL; with permission.)

process or have grown to a size for which reconstruction will be useful. This is particularly helpful for patients with microtia who must wait until at least 5 to 7 years of age before the contralateral ear is of adult size. For other areas, such as orbital reconstruction, surgery simply cannot replace the lost tissues.

In addition, prosthetics are often overlooked as an adjunct to surgical reconstruction. Prosthetics contribute to a protective barrier of sensitive tissues during the healing process. Prosthodontics provide functional components by closing oral fistulas and providing teeth for oral eating either temporarily or permanently.

Prosthetics can be a part of optimal medical management. Patients who need postoperative radiation therapy benefit from a temporary prosthesis that can be removed for treatment (**Fig. 4**). This leaves the tumor bed unobscured by tissue flaps, and reconstruction can occur at a later date using healthy nonradiated tissue. In addition, removable prosthetics can facilitate tumor surveillance during the most high-risk period for recurrence, typically the first year after treatment completion.[22]

Types of Implants

Facial prosthetics may be categorized based on how they are applied. The simplest implants are anatomically retained, fitting into existing anatomic structures or cavities. Others are mechanically retained, attaching to another removable object such as eye glasses. Some types may also require adhesive for attachment, which must be cleaned and reapplied daily. The most long-lasting and secure are implant-retained prosthetics that attach to titanium endosseous implants that may be placed in native or irradiated bone.[23] In reality, a prosthetic may use one or more retention types for the best final appearance.

The surgical defect dictates the implant characteristics; therefore, early communication between the surgeon and the prosthetics team is important. A good implant surface has thin, fixed, hairless tissue overlying bone or cartilage. Split-thickness skin graft coverage of the resection cavities is ideal (**Fig. 5**). Filling in of cavity defects with soft tissue flaps is not required. Because the prosthesis works as an occlusive dressing, sinus cavities can be left open. In fact, implants are easier to

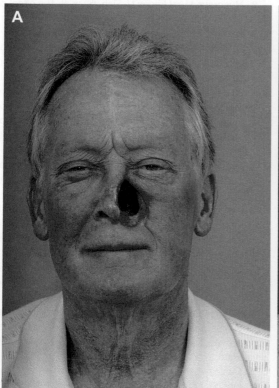
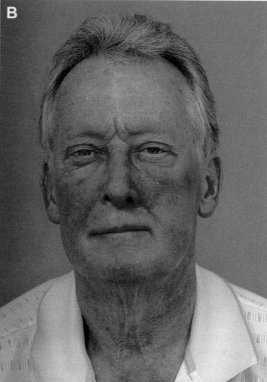

Fig. 4. A lateral nasal and sinus defect after sarcoma removal (*A*) with a temporary nasal prosthesis (*B*) designed to be removed for radiation therapy and tumor surveillance with delayed surgical reconstruction. (Prosthesis fabricated by anaplastologist Rosemary Seelaus.) (*Courtesy of* The Craniofacial Center, University of Illinois at Chicago, Chicago, IL; with permission.)

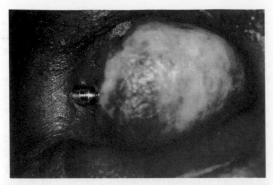

Fig. 5. An ideal ocular cavity showing the endosseous titanium implant for attachment and demonstrating a large cavity with thin, fixed, hairless skin. (Prosthesis fabricated by anaplastologist Michaela Calhoun.) (*Courtesy of* The Craniofacial Center, University of Illinois at Chicago, Chicago, IL; with permission.)

design and adhere better if a cavity remains, even in large defects. Anatomic retention principles can be incorporated into the implant, making it easier to apply with less need for adhesive or fine manipulation. This may be an important lifestyle consideration for children or the elderly.

The expectations of patients using prosthetics must be realistic. Just as with surgical reconstruction, prosthetics are not native form. They are insensate and immobile; the tissues will never exactly match the surrounding facial form. These prosthetics also require daily application and upkeep. However, they provide an important nonsurgical alternative for coverage of maxillofacial defects, allowing scar camouflage and return to daily life in patients.

SUMMARY

Patients have increasing expectations for scar appearance, and facial plastic surgeons are an integral part of scar management. However, significant scar camouflage can be achieved without surgery. Minimization of scar formation begins with good wound care, including moisturizing and minimization of trauma. Although silicone and vitamin A have been shown to improve scar appearance, other topical agents, such as biological extracts and vitamin E, have minimal benefit. Pressure dressings are helpful particularly with burn scars; scar massage may help pruritis but has not been shown to greatly improve scar appearance alone. As a result, cosmetics have been developed to be particularly helpful in scar camouflage. In addition, patients have a range of hairstyling and use of glasses that detracts from facial scars. Facial prosthetics should be

considered for large defects or those in whom tumor treatment or surveillance would benefit from delayed repair.

REFERENCES

1. Tebble NJ, Adams R, Thomas DW, et al. Anxiety and self-consciousness in patients with facial lacerations one week and six months later. Br J Oral Maxillofac Surg 2006;44(6):520–5.
2. Brown BC, McKenna SP, Siddhi K, et al. The hidden cost of skin scars: quality of life after skin scarring. J Plast Reconstr Aesthet Surg 2008;61(9):1049–58.
3. Chang CW, Ries WR. Nonoperative techniques for scar management and revision. Facial Plast Surg 2001;17(4):283–8.
4. Goldberg SR, Dieglemann RF. Wound healing primer. Surg Clin North Am 2010;90(6):1133–46.
5. Ogawa R. The most current algorithms for the treatment and prevention of hypertrophic scars and keloids. Plast Reconstr Surg 2010;125(2):557–68.
6. Eaglestein WH. Experiences with biosynthetic dressings. J Am Acad Dermatol 1985;12:434.
7. Suetak T, Sasai S, Zhen YX, et al. Effects of silicone get sheet on the stratum corneum hydration. Br J Plast Surg 2000;53:503–7.
8. Musgrave MA, Umraw N, Fish JS, et al. The effect of silicone gel sheets on perfusion of hypertrophic burn scars. J Burn Care Rehabil 2002;23(3):208–14.
9. Bianchi FA, Roccia F, Fiorini P, et al. Use of Patient and Observer Scar Assessment Scale for evaluation of facial scars treated with self-drying silicone gel. J Craniofac Surg 2010;21(3):719–23.
10. Signorini M, Clementoni MT. Clinical evaluation of a new self-drying silicone gel in the treatment of scars: a preliminary report. Aesthetic Plast Surg 2007;31(2):183–7.
11. Janssen de Limpens AM. The local treatment of hypertrophic scars and keloids with topical retinoic acid. Br J Dermatol 1980;103(3):319–23.
12. Jenkins M, Alexander JW, MacMillan BG, et al. Failure of topical steroids and vitamin E to reduce postoperative scar formation following reconstructive surgery. J Burn Care Rehabil 1986;7:309–12.
13. Baumann LS, Spencer J. The effects of topical vitamin E on the cosmetic appearance of scars. Dermatol Surg 1999;25:311–5.
14. Chung VQ, Kelley L, Marra D, et al. Onion extract gel versus petrolatum emollient on new surgical scars: prospective double-blinded study. Dermatol Surg 2006;32(2):193–7.
15. Costa AM, Peyrol S, Porto LC, et al. Mechanical forces induce scar remodeling: study in non-pressure-treated versus pressure-treated hypertrophic scars. Am J Pathol 1999;155:1671–9.
16. Roh YS, Cho H, Oh JO, et al. Effects of skin rehabilitation massage therapy on pruritis, skin status, and

depression in burn survivors. Taechan Kanho Hakhoe Chi 2007;37(2):221–6.

17. Patino O, Novick C, Merlo A, et al. Massage in hypertrophic scars. J Burn Care Rehabil 1999;20:267–71.

18. Tedeschi A, Dall'Oglio F, Micali G, et al. Corrective camouflage in pediatric dermatology. Cutis 2007; 79(2):110–2.

19. Roberts NC. Corrective cosmetics—need, evaluation and use. Cutis 1988;41(6):439–41.

20. Fiedler JG. Foundation makeup. Cosmetics: science and technology. 2nd edition. New York: John Wiley & Sons; 1972. p. 317.

21. Meyer-Marcotty P, Gerdes A, Stellzig-Eisenhauer A, et al. Visual face perception of adults with unilateral cleft lip and palate in comparison to controls—an eye tracking study. Cleft Palate Craniofac J 2011; 48(2):210–6.

22. Reisberg DJ. Maxillofacial prosthetics: rehabilitation of the head and neck cancer patient. Ill Dent J 1988; 57(5):346–9.

23. Visser A, Raghoebar GM, van Oort RP, et al. Fate of implant-retained craniofacial prostheses: life span and aftercare. Int J Oral Maxillofac Implants 2008; 23(1):89–98.

Proper Care of Early Wounds to Optimize Healing and Prevent Complications

Geoffrey B. Pitzer, MD, Krishna G. Patel, MD, PhD*

KEYWORDS

- Wounds • Wound complications • Wound healing
- Contaminated wounds • Avulsed wounds

The proverb states, "time heals all wounds" and, fortunately, through the resilience of the human body, this often holds true. As medicine advances, so has understanding of the mechanisms of wound healing. Elucidation of the healing process has permitted better opportunities to promote healing while minimizing scar formation. We possess a gross understanding of the key cells and factors that manipulate healing; however, the ability to translate this knowledge into clinical use is still lacking and limits the potential to completely control and enhance the process.

Surgery inherently implies the creation of a wound and, consequently, all wounds create scar. Therefore, an important and unspoken goal in surgery is to accomplish the procedure while minimizing scar formation. Proper surgical techniques for wound closure have long been described, and through continued affirmation, these concepts have evolved into tenets rather than mere recommendations.

Wound healing is important in a wide range of scenarios, whether a patient is healing from a chronic open ulcer or healing from a planned scar revision. The ability to optimize the early care of wounds can greatly aid in the expediency of a wound healing, as well as in the final aesthetic appearance. Although there is no absolute way to care for a wound, this article describes key points that can aid in promoting improved healing while preventing future complications, such as the development of a chronic wound, a hypertrophic scar, or a visibly undesirable scar.

WOUND HEALING PHASES

Understanding the basic stages of wound healing is imperative to best regulate the process. The physiology of wound healing involves multiple phases over time and can be organized into the following phases (**Fig. 1**):

- Inflammatory
- Proliferative
- Remodeling/maturation.

Inflammatory Phase

During the initial injury, hemostasis is of primary importance, and immediate vasoconstriction occurs. Vasoconstriction is mediated by thromboxane A_2 and lasts for 5 to 10 minutes.[1] Endothelial cell injury and exposure of collagen, fibronectin, and laminin lead to activation of the coagulation and complement cascades, which initiate the formation of a clot consisting of fibrin and aggregated platelets.[2] Activated platelets release prostaglandins and vasoactive materials, such as serotonin, histamine, proteases, and thromboxane, which go on to activate their target cells (**Box 1**).

After initial vasoconstriction, active vasodilation occurs, likely secondary to histamine release from mast cells and circulating serotonin. Subsequently,

Department of Otolaryngology – Head and Neck Surgery, Medical University of South Carolina, 135 Rutledge Avenue, Charleston, SC 29425, USA
* Corresponding author.
E-mail address: patelkg@musc.edu

Facial Plast Surg Clin N Am 19 (2011) 491–504
doi:10.1016/j.fsc.2011.06.012
1064-7406/11/$ – see front matter

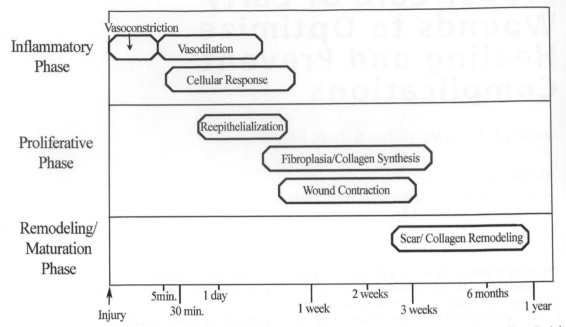

Fig. 1. Phases of wound healing. (*Adapted from* Fisher E, Frodel JL. Wound healing. In: Papel ID, editor. Facial plastic and reconstructive surgery. 3rd edition. New York: Thieme; 2009; with permission.)

kallikrein is activated, leading to kinin activation and endothelial cell separation, which then allows increased vascular permeability that continues for the first 48 to 72 hours.[3]

The cellular response in the inflammatory phase lags somewhat behind the vascular changes, and it begins as fibronectin promotes the migration of neutrophils, monocytes, fibroblasts, and endothelial cells into the region of injury.[2] Fibronectin forms cross-links with clot, which epithelial cells and fibroblasts use as a temporary matrix to proliferate in the wound.[4] Polymorphonuclear leukocytes (granulocytes) and monocytes are among the first cells to appear after an injury. Stimulated by chemotactic factors, granulocytes appear within 6 hours of an insult, and act to clean the wound by phagocytic removal of bacteria and debris. In a noncontaminated wound, the presence of granulocytes is generally short-lived; however, in a contaminated wound, granulocytes can persist and prolong the inflammatory phase. Lengthened periods of inflammation may account for worsened scarring.[2]

Macrophages are essential for wound healing by providing a critical regulatory function in the inflammatory phase and by transitioning a wound into a stage of repair. Attracted by platelet-derived growth factor (PDGF), macrophages are the predominant cell type in a wound by 48 to 96 hours.[1] Macrophages release chemotactic and growth factors, such as transforming growth factor β (TGF-β), basic fibroblast growth factor (FGF), epidermal growth factor, transforming growth factor-α (TGF-α),

and PDGF, that result in endothelial and fibroblast proliferation[2] (**Table 1**). If macrophage function is diminished, granulation tissue formation, fibroplasia, collagen production, and, subsequently, overall wound healing, are decreased.[5] The immune response is also closely linked to wound repair, because lymphocytes produce important factors, such as TGF-β, interferons, interleukins, and tumor necrosis factor, that interact with macrophages.[6]

As wound inflammation subsides, collagen deposition can begin, resulting in increased wound tensile strength. Wound strength early in the inflammatory phase is minimal and based on fibrin clot and early epithelialization.[7] At the end of the inflammatory phase, approximately 5 to 7 days after injury, a wound has only approximately 10% of its final tensile strength.[2]

Proliferative Phase

The proliferative phase is the next major step in wound healing, and it is characterized by:

- Re-epithelialization
- Neovascularization
- Collagen deposition
- Wound contraction.

Re-epithelialization begins within 24 hours of injury as epithelial cells from wound margins or deeper adnexal structures, such as hair follicles or sebaceous glands, migrate into the wound to re-establish a protective barrier over underlying

> **Box 1**
> **Substances released from platelets after injury**
>
> Substances Released From α Granules of Platelets During Wound Healing
>
> Platelet-derived growth factor
>
> Basic fibroblast growth factor
>
> Vascular endothelial growth factor
>
> Transforming growth factor β1
>
> Transforming growth factor α
>
> Epidermal growth factor
>
> Thrombospondin
>
> Platelet thromboplastin
>
> Coagulation factors
>
> Serotonin
>
> Histamine
>
> Platelet-activating factor
>
> Hydrolytic enzymes
>
> Endostatin (antiangiogenic)
>
> *Data from* Hom DB, Sun GH, Ravindra GE. A contemporary review of wound healing in otolaryngology: current state and future promise. Laryngoscope 2009;119:2099–110.

tissues.[2] Granulation tissue develops approximately 3 to 4 days after an injury, and it is composed of inflammatory cells, new blood vessels, and fibroblasts in a matrix containing fibrin, glycoproteins, collagen, and glycosaminoglycans.[8] Granulation tissue serves as a scaffold for cell migration, and it is present until re-epithelialization is complete.[2] Re-epithelialization occurs rapidly in wounds closed primarily but can take 3 to 5 days in a wound healing by secondary intention.[3] A moist environment aids the movement of epithelial cells, with most rapid wound coverage occurring in occluded moist wounds. In contrast, migrating epithelium takes longer over desiccated or partially necrotic surfaces, leading to significantly impaired wound healing (**Fig. 2**).[9]

Fibroblasts are a critical cellular element in a healing wound's proliferative phase. These cells generally appear approximately 2 to 3 days after an injury, and they replicate and migrate in response to mediators, including C5a, fibronectin, PDGF, FGF, and TGF-β.[10] Fibroblasts are involved in the production of collagen, elastin, fibronectin, glycosaminoglycans, and collagenase, which is important in the later maturation and remodeling phase of wound healing.[11] Collagen synthesis increases dramatically by the fourth day after an injury. Fibroblasts secrete procollagen that is cleaved to tropocollagen, which then aggregates into fibrils that combine to form the collagen fiber, where subsequent cross-linking aids in increasing local tissue strength. Type III collagen predominates in early wound healing, but type I collagen is the major component in mature scar tissue.

Wound contraction, also an integral component of the proliferative phase of wound healing, is mediated by myofibroblasts, which are differentiated fibroblasts. Maximal contraction occurs at 12 to 15 days at an average of 0.6 to 0.75 mm of movement a day.[1] Contraction of a wound becomes more severe if there is significant inflammation present or if the wound is left open for an extended period.[2] Wound contraction is lessened in the presence of skin grafts, but it is still significant, with full-thickness skin grafts commonly experiencing 20% contraction.[12]

Remodeling/Maturation Phase

The final stage of wound healing is the remodeling or maturation phase. Type III collagen is gradually replaced by type I collagen, and the maturing scar becomes stronger while also decreasing in size and erythema. Further organization of collagen fibers into a more parallel fashion allows for increased tensile strength and an improved appearance. The neovascularization of the wound eventually regresses, leading to a relatively avascular mature scar. Final remodeling of a wound may take 12 to 18 months, and the scar will have, at maximum, 70% to 80% of the original tensile strength of healthy, unwounded skin.[2]

CLINICAL CONSIDERATIONS/DISEASES THAT IMPEDE HEALING

The physiology of optimal wound healing can be adversely affected by both local and systemic factors (**Table 2**). Local factors having an impact on healing include[2]

- Wound closure techniques
- Wound dessication
- Tissue ischemia
- Local infection.

Many chronic medical conditions can result in suboptimal or impaired wound healing because of poor nutrition or immunologic function[2]:

- Vascular conditions
- Metabolic disorders
- Immune deficiency states
- Chronic liver disease
- Diabetes mellitus
- Malignancies
- Thrombocytopenic conditions.

Table 1
Cytokines involved in wound healing

Cytokine	Abbreviation	Source	Function
Human growth hormone	GH	Pituitary gland	Fibroblast proliferation; increases collagen content and tensile strength; anabolism; stimulates IFG-1
Epidermal growth factor	EGF	Platelets, bodily fluids	Epithelial cell and fibroblast proliferation and migration; activates fibroblasts; angiogenic
Platelet-derived growth factor	PDGF	Platelets, macrophages, fibroblasts, endothelial cells, smooth muscle cells	Mitogenic for fibroblasts and smooth muscle cells; chemoattractant for neutrophils and macrophages; angiogenic
Fibroblast growth factor	FGF	Macrophages, brain, pituitary gland	Proliferation and migration of vascular endothelial cells; mitogenic and chemotactic for keratinocytes and fibroblasts
Transforming growth factor	TGF	Platelets, fibroblasts, neutrophils, macrophages, lymphocytes	Epithelial cell and fibroblast factors proliferation
Insulinlike growth factor 1	IGF-1	Fibroblasts, liver, plasma	Fibroblast proliferation; proteoglycan and collagen synthesis
Tumor necrosis factor	TNF	Macrophages, mast cells, lymphocytes, other tissues and cells	Fibroblast proliferation
Interleukins	ILs	Macrophages, lymphocytes, other tissues and cells	Fibroblast proliferation; neutrophil chemotaxis
Interferons	IFNs	Fibroblasts, lymphocytes	Inhibition of fibroblast proliferation and collagen synthesis
Keratinocyte growth factors	KGFs	Fibroblasts	Epithelial cell proliferation

Data from Terris DJ. Dynamics in wound healing. In: Bailey BJ, editor. Head and neck surgery—otolaryngology. Philadelphia: Lippincott-Raven; 1998.

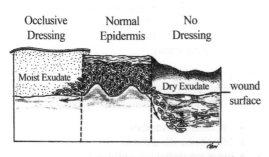

Fig. 2. Rapid epithelialization is promoted with moist occlusion and slowed under dried clot. (*Adapted from* Fisher E, Frodel JL. Wound healing. In: Papel ID, editor. Facial plastic and reconstructive surgery. 3rd edition. New York: Thieme; 2009; with permission.)

Although more rare, systemic genetic disorders, such as Ehlers-Danlos syndrome, cutis laxa, osteogenesis imperfecta, and progeria, can alter normal healing mechanisms. In addition, congenital errors in metabolism that result in defective collagen production have an impact on the later phases of wound healing.

Advanced age results in slower healing and decreased wound tensile strength.[13] History of radiation therapy is also a known risk factor for poor wound healing. Systemic medications can have a significant clinical impact on the healing process. Corticosteroids inhibit aspects of the inflammatory phase and diminish collagen synthesis and wound contraction. Corticosteroids also decrease cellular defense mechanisms, resulting in increased infection risk.[14] Similarly, certain chemotherapeutic medications can affect wound healing by altering the inflammatory response, collagen synthesis, or wound contraction.[15]

Table 2
Factors that impair normal wounding healing

Systemic Factors	Local Factors
Hereditary	Ischemia
• Coagulation disorders	Infection
• Ehlers-Danlos/Marfan	Tissue trauma
• Prolidase deficiency	Retained foreign
• Werner syndromes	body desiccation
Vascular disorders	Medications
• Congestive heart	Glucocorticoids
failure	Anticoagulants
• Atherosclerosis	Antineoplastic agents
• Hypertension	Colchicine
• Vasculitis	Penicillamine
• Venous stasis	Vitamin E
• Lymphedema	Salicylates
Metabolic	(high dose)
• Chronic renal failure	Nonsteroidals
• Diabetes mellitus	(high dose)
• Malnutrition	Zinc sulfate
• Cushing syndromes	(high dose)
• Hyper/hypothyroidism	Vitamin A
Immunologic	(high dose)
deficiency states	
Chronic pulmonary	
disease	
Liver failure	
Malignancy	

Data from Terris DJ. Dynamics in wound healing. In: Bailey BJ, editor. Head and neck surgery—otolaryngology. Philadelphia: Lippincott-Raven; 1998.

CREATING THE OPTIMAL ENVIRONMENT FOR HEALING
Nutrition

The process of healing places the body into an anabolic state that requires additional energy intake; therefore, the first step to improving healing conditions should begin with assessing the health of the patient. Serum albumin is an essential tool in assessing nutritional status. The Veterans Administration cooperative study of preoperative risk factors and adverse outcomes linked low serum albumin levels to increased risk for wound dehiscence or wound complications.[16] These findings emphasize the need for adequate essential amino acid supply and protein synthesis. Deficiency in protein synthesis has been recognized as delaying healing through suppression of fibroblast proliferation, angiogenesis, collagen synthesis, and collagen remodeling.[17]

Although providing supplemental nutrition for diseased or malnourished patients to improve healing is commonplace, few studies have examined the effects of nutritional supplementation on wound healing in healthy individuals. A randomized

controlled crossover trial that provided an oral vitamin supplement (containing proteases, bromelain, vitamin C, calcium, rutin [bioflavanoids], and grapeseed extract) revealed accelerated healing in the supplemented patient group when compared with the control group. Although the study suggested more rapid healing, no comment was made on the final aesthetic outcome of the scar.[18] These data support the concept that several vitamins play essential roles in proper healing. Vitamin A is important for the cross-linking and synthesis of collagen, with deficiencies causing inhibition of epithelialization and delayed wound closure.[3] Likewise, vitamin C is required for the proper hydroxylation of proline and lysine during collagen cross-linking. Without this hydroxylation step, the collagen molecule would be unstable, providing no tensile strength and little resistance to enzymatic breakdown.[17] Vitamin C also serves an important role in neutrophil function as a reducing agent in superoxide radical formation.[2,18] The vitamin B family also participates in collagen cross-linking. Zinc is involved in the enzymatic activity of RNA and DNA synthesis and collagenase function. Deficiencies in zinc cause delays in epithelialization and fibroblast formation.[19] In contrast, vitamin E has been shown to reduce collagen production and tensile strength. For this reason, vitamin E has become a popular topical cream to prevent scar hypertrophy, although there is lacking statistical evidence that application of vitamin E actually improves scars. Although there are no definitive studies proving that supplementation of vitamins enhances healing in healthy individuals, there are data that vitamin deficiencies have a negative impact on the healing process. For this reason, the nutritional status of a patient should always be assessed, especially in the setting of a poorly healing wound.

Cleaning Agents/Cleaning Wounds

When selecting a wound cleaner, its cleaning capacity must be weighed against the potential toxicity of the cleaning agent to the cells within the wound bed. The utility of antiseptics on intact skin is well established and broadly accepted; however, the application of antiseptics to open wounds, especially those containing detergents, has been controversial secondary to potential cytotoxic effects on fibroblasts, keratinocytes, and leukocytes within the wound.[20–22]

Hydrogen peroxide is a popular antiseptic cleansing agent, but its use in open wounds continues to be controversial. A review of the literature evaluating both in vitro and in vivo studies revealed that although 3% hydrogen peroxide had low toxicity on tissues, it showed poor ability to reduce the bacterial load within wounds. This review concluded that hydrogen peroxide is safe for use in open wounds and may provide some mechanical benefit in loosening debris and necrotic tissue, but it may be inefficient as an antiseptic.[23]

One of the most common agents used in wound cleaning is 0.9% sodium chloride (saline). It is widely accepted as a gentle means for cleansing all types of wounds. Additionally, a Cochrane collaboration study suggested water, although not isotonic, is an acceptable alternative method to saline.[24] (Cochrane studies are systematic reviews performed by health care providers that analyze primary research publications to objectively provide evidenced-based decisions on a particular topic. The Cochrane Collaboration, a nonprofit organization that is independent from financial interests, upholds a nonbiased opinion on an evaluated topic.)

In the setting of contaminated wounds, multiple methods for washing out debris have been described, including high-pressure pulsed lavage irrigations and bulb syringe irrigations. When compared directly, high-pressure pulsed lavage irrigation demonstrated superior results in the removal of contaminants.[25] Irrigation pressures of 10 psi and 15 psi are more effective at removing bacteria and debris than 1 psi and 5 psi.[26] Irrigation pressures of 20 psi or greater did not show increased efficacy and raised concern about potentially causing penetration of debris deeper into the wound. Regardless of the method of irrigation delivery, copious amounts of irrigant should be used to remove contaminants and bacteria. Irrigants commonly used include saline or antibiotic-infused saline (such as 50,000 units of bacitracin to 1 L of saline).

Surgical Techniques for Optimizing Wound Healing

To optimize wound healing, several guidelines exist to direct the proper employment of surgical technique (**Box 2**). These include the tenets set forth by renown surgeon Dr William Stewart Halsted[7]:

1. Gentle handling of tissue
2. Aseptic technique
3. Sharp anatomic dissection of tissue
4. Careful hemostasis
5. Obliteration of dead space
6. Avoidance of tension
7. Reliance on rest.

Additional key points include[27]:

1. Removal of necrotic tissue and foreign bodies
2. Control and prevention of infection

Box 2
Tenets of wound care

Surgical technique

> Aseptic technique
> Gentle handling of tissue
> Sharp anatomic dissection of tissue
> Obliterate dead space
> Maintain hemostasis
> Remove necrotic tissue and foreign bodies
> Freshen wound edges
> Avoid tension on wound edges

Tissue management

> Control and prevention of infection
> Absorb excess exudates/divert secretions/use drains when appropriate
> Maintain a moist environment to promote granulation and re-epithelialization

---

3. Diversion of salivary secretions
4. Absorption of excess exudates with the use of drains when necessary
5. Creation of fresh wound edges to promote re-epithelialization
6. Coverage with skin grafts or flaps when appropriate.

Adherence to these principles prevents the conversion of an acute wound into a chronic wound and improve the ultimate cosmetic results of the scar. For example, both hypertrophic and atrophic scars can directly result from poor handling of tissues and excessive tension on wound edges (**Table 3**). With respect to aesthetics, additional consideration should be placed on the location of any planned incisions. Making incisions along relaxed skin tension lines allows wounds to be closed along the vectors of maximal extensibility, serving to minimize tension and camouflage the incision within natural skin creases. Additionally, although removal of necrotic tissue is advocated, aggressive excision of tissue is not recommended in either primary or delayed treatment.[17]

When considering the final scar appearance, suture materials used for the wound closure must be considered for their potential impact on cosmesis. Ideally, the most nonreactive and smallest caliber suture should be used with good tissue eversion. A meta-analysis comparing permanent suture versus absorbable suture concluded that there is a need for better randomized controlled studies to infer any difference in cosmetic outcomes.[28] Selection of wound closure material

Table 3
Complications in wound healing

Complications	Means to Prevent Complications
Acute complications	
Infection	• Aseptic technique • Copious irrigation of contaminated wounds
Necrosis	• HBO treatments
Wound dehiscence	• Avoid excess tension on wound closure • Prevent infection, hematoma, or seroma within wound
Poor healing	• Multifactorial • Assess patient health
Chronic complications	
Hyperpigmented scar	• Apply sun protection agents • Avoid prolonged inflammation during the healing period
Hypopigmented scar	• Avoid excessive steroid injections • Avoid excess tension on wound closure
Nonhealing wound	• Multifactorial • Assess patient health
Hypertrophic scar	• Avoid excess tension on wound closure • Avoid prolonged inflammation during the healing period
Atrophic scar	• Avoid excess tension on wound closure
Visibly undesirable scar	• Design incisions within relaxed skin tension lines
Keloid	• Multifactorial • Avoid excess tension on wound closure

facial lacerations.[29] This review applied only to linear wounds less than 4 cm. There was a statistically significant difference in wound dehiscence between use of sutures and tissue glue in the Cochrane study, with the risk difference of 2.4%. Similarly, a randomized controlled study comparing Steri-strips to tissue glue, Dermabond, demonstrated comparable results between the two methods of closure, although the evaluation period was for 2 months only.[30]

Moist Environment/Dressings

Substantial evidence supports the importance of maintaining a moist environment for healing wounds. In the scenario of a surgically closed wound, epithelialization is completed within 24 to 48 hours; however, in an open wound, the re-epithelialization process takes much longer. Maintaining moist conditions during this period allows direct and unimpeded migration of epithelial cells. In the setting of a desiccated and crusted open wound, migration is less efficient and proceeds along a less direct route, thus delaying wound closure (see **Fig. 2**).

Studies suggest that a moist wound bed may increase the rate of epithelialization by twofold.[27] Thus, it is important for occlusive or semiocclusive dressings to create a moist environment while wicking away excess fluid, because seromas and hematomas are known to impede wound healing.[17,31] Ideally, a balance can be created between maintaining a moist environment yet preventing excessive moisture that leads to maceration of intact surrounding skin or the promotion of bacterial growth. Fortunately, several options exist for selecting the appropriate dressing. Different dressings may have multiple properties that must be taken into account based on the specific needs of the wound.[32] **Table 4** briefly describes a variety of occlusive dressing options and their properties (see **Table 4**).

Topical Wound Products

Many topical agents have been used to maintain appropriate wound moisture, including petrolatum ointments, water-based gels, and antibiotic ointments. Antibiotic topical creams have the dual purpose of moisturizing and preventing infection, although many studies have questioned the need for antibiotic ointments in a clean wound.[33] The incidence of allergic contact dermatitis has been reported as high as 7.8% to 13.1% for bacitracin ointments and 34% for Neosporin.[2,34] A randomized double-blinded prospective trial that compared white petrolatum to bacitracin in 922 individuals revealed no statistically significant

can vary significantly depending on the scenario. For example, incisions in children are often closed with absorbable suture to avoid the need for subsequent suture removal. Likewise, many studies demonstrate the use of nonsuture materials, such as tissue glues and Steri-strips, in emergency medicine. A Cochrane review of randomized controlled trials evaluating the use of tissue glues versus sutures suggested the cosmetic outcome of each type of closure as comparable, although only one of the examined studies was specific to

Table 4
Types of surgical dressings

Class	Composition	Examples	Adhesive	Absorbent	Gas Permeable	Fluid Permeable	Uses
Gauze	Cotton fiber	Gauze	−	+	+	+	Nonspecific débriding action, drying, variety of wounds
Impregnated gauze	Cotton fiber + antibiotic agent	Xeroform	−	±	+	+	Maintains wound moisture, variety of wounds
Adhesive films	Polyurethane	OpSite, Tegaderm, Bioclusive	+	−	+	−	Sutured wounds, Cutaneous ulcers, skin graft sites; poor for wounds with heavy exudates
Hydrogels	Water + hydrophilic copolymer	Hydrogel	−	−	+	−	Cutaneous ulcers, maintains wound moisture, poor for wounds with heavy exudates
Hydrocolloids	Colloids	Duoderm	+	+	−	−	Cutaneous ulcers, poor for wounds with heavy exudates
Foams	Polyurethane based	Lyofoam	−	+	+	+	Absorbs moderate amounts of exudates, hydrophilic
Silicone based	Silicone	Biobrane, Mepiform	±	−	+	−	Cutaneous ulcers, hypertrophic scars
Bioengineered skin	Cultured keratinocytes or fibroblasts	Apligraf, Transcyte, Epicel, Dermagraft, Integra (collagen)	−	Variable	+	+	Full-thickness ulcers or burns

differences in postprocedural infections (2% with petrolatum and 0.9% with bacitracin), contact dermatitis (0% for petrolatum and 0.9% for bacitracin), or healing between the two groups.[33]

A prospective randomized study that compared patient wound healing using a topical antibiotic, moist exposed burn ointment, or open air reported significantly improved cosmetic appearance of the scar with use of moist exposed burn ointment.[35] Noncompliance was a large concern, however, with the product secondary to its oily and fragrant properties. This study was unique in that it assessed the aesthetic qualities of the final wound.

Antiscar Agents

Once the wound has closed, the next phase of wound care shifts to prevention of excessive healing, or hypertrophy. This is a popular topic of debate and many existing over-the-counter products tout antiscar properties. Steroid injections have long been the mainstay of treatment for reducing inflammation within a wound during healing periods and for prevention of hypertrophic scarring.[36,37] The postulated mechanism of action of steroid injections is the reduction of fibroblast proliferation and collagen synthesis as well as suppression of inflammatory mediators and glycosaminoglycan synthesis.[38] In the setting of hypertrophic scars, one study reported intralesional injection of triamcinolone acetonide led to symptomatic improvement in 72% of patients and complete flattening in 64% of lesions.[39,40] Steroid injections should avoid penetration into the surrounding tissue to prevent complications, such as atrophy, hypopigmentation, and telangiectasia.

A popular antiscar topical product is the onion extract, Mederma. The active ingredient in Mederma is a derivative of quercetin, a bioflavonoid. It is speculated as having antiproliferative and antiinflammatory properties.[31] In a rabbit model study there was no statistically significant difference in the physical appearance of scars treated with Mederma compared with control groups; however, histologic evaluation suggested improved collagen organization in the Mederma-treated experimental group.[41] Similarly, a randomized double-blind study in humans comparing healing outcomes using Mederma to petrolatum suggested no statistical difference in wound healing between the two topical agents.[42]

Since the 1980s, a wide range of silicone-based products has been used in the treatment of hypertrophic scars and keloids. Review of the literature reveals that the application of silicone gel has shown improvements in redness, itching, texture, and thickness of hypertrophic scars and keloids

in a majority of patients. Silicone creates a water-impermeable plastic film, thus acting as another protective layer of skin and also serving to hydrate scar tissue. Silicone also reduces the activity of mast cells, the level of interleukin 1, and extracellular matrix production, all leading to decreased collagen synthesis.[43]

Self-drying silicone gel has demonstrated satisfactory healing in surgical and posttraumatic facial scars, and it is especially useful on sedated patients and in children, where massage of facial scars may be difficult.[44] Similarly, Hydrogel sheeting has been approved by the Food and Drug Administration as equivalent to silicone for the treatment of hypertrophic scars.[45]

In addition to topical medicines, pressure dressings were observed by Larson and colleagues[46] as helpful in the management of scar hypertrophy. Subsequently, pressure dressings of 20 to 204 mm Hg have become a favorable technique used for scar prevention.[45] When pressure dressings are not feasible, massage of the wound can mimic the effects of a pressure dressing.

Protection of fresh wounds or scars from sun exposure is imperative for optimal wound healing. Hyperpigmentation may result after sun exposure to recently epithelialized and fragile healing skin. This complication is best avoided with the use of topical sunblock for the first year on a newly healed wound.[47]

Negative Pressure Wound Therapy

Vacuum-assisted negative pressure dressings have demonstrated their utility in the management of open wounds and skin graft care (**Fig. 3**). Use of negative pressure wound therapy stimulates granulation tissue formation, decreases bacterial load, increases blood flow, stimulates neovascularization, and reduces edema.[48] Negative pressure vacuum-assisted devices have been used successfully in split-thickness and full-thickness skin grafting as well as in degloving injuries of the hand and foot.[49] These devices show benefit particularly in the healing of split-thickness skin grafts on irregular surfaces where traditional bolsters are difficult to secure. Along irregular surfaces, negative pressure vacuum-assisted devices have demonstrated a 95% take rate with split-thickness skin grafts.[50]

Hyperbaric Oxygen Therapy

As wounds become more challenging, higher levels of technology, such as negative pressure vacuum-assisted devices and hyperbaric oxygen (HBO) therapy, display their utility. HBO treatments typically apply pressures of 2 to 3 atmospheres

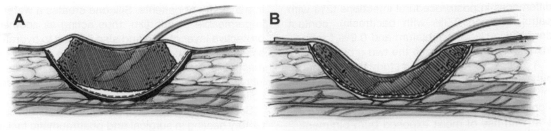

Fig. 3. (*A*) Vacuum-assisted device sponge over skin graft. (*B*) Vacuum-assisted device sponge with negative pressure applied. (*Adapted from* Hom DB, Sun GH, Ravindra GE. A contemporary review of wound healing in otolaryngology: current state and future promise. Laryngoscope 2009;119:2099–110; with permission.)

absolute for 1.5 to 2.0 hours per treatment. Usually, treatments are administered once to twice daily for 20 to 40 treatments. The potential advantages of HBO therapy include increased neovascularization and increased oxygen tissue diffusion, both of which improve oxygen delivery to hypoxic areas of wounds.[51–53] Although HBO therapy has gained acceptance for treatment of bodily wounds, there exist few data for its use in the head and neck region. Guidelines set forth by the Undersea and Hyperbaric Medical Society recommend HBO therapy for crush/traumatic ischemic injuries, compromised grafts and flaps, and delayed complications from radiation therapy as well as for enhancement of healing in selected problem wounds. Of these indications, most of the published literature supports HBO treatments for healing chronic diabetic wounds and treatments of osteoradionecrosis.

A few case reports suggest facilitated tissue survival in the setting of near avulsion or degloving injuries in the face.[54,55] With respect to timing, one study evaluated healing of surgical flaps in previously radiated soft tissue and concluded that patients who underwent preoperative and postoperative HBO therapy were reported to have better healing with less complication when compare with patients who received postoperative HBO therapy or no HBO therapy. Specifically, the study had a total of 36 patients: 75% of 23 patients treated with preoperative and postoperative HBO therapy healed without major complication, 25% of 19 patients treated with only postoperative HBO therapy healed without major complication, and 0% of 6 patients treated with no HBO therapy healed without major complication.[56] Additionally, there seems to be an advantage to initiating HBO therapy in the immediate perioperative period compared with delaying treatments for salvage efforts.

Complications reported for HBO include a rare (1 in 10,000 patients) risk of grand mal seizure from central nervous system oxygen toxicity, reversible progressive myopia, and nuclear cataracts with excessive HBO treatments. A common

risk for HBO therapy is otologic barotrauma, with a range of 14% to 30% of patients requiring pressure equalization tubes to prevent otologic complications. The benefits of HBO therapy seem promising for use within the head and neck region, but more clinical analysis and research data are warranted to better understand the benefits.[53]

Botulinum Toxin Type A

Novel uses for botulinum toxin have also been examined for healing purposes. Tension acting on wound edges during healing is an important factor in determining the final cosmetic appearance of a scar. The use of botulinum toxin for chemoimmobilization of facial wounds has been shown to be safe; however, delayed onset of muscle inactivity is a shortcoming.[57] Therefore, chemoimmobilization is most useful in an anticipated surgical procedure where the injection can be performed 1 to 2 weeks before the procedure. In a blinded, prospective, randomized clinical trial, botulinum toxin–induced immobilization of forehead wounds enhanced healing and resulted in less noticeable scars.[58] Researchers have also shown that local injection of botulinum toxin can inhibit the formation of hypertrophic scar and the activity of fibroblasts in the rabbit ear model.[59] It is suggested that botulinum toxin decreases the expression of collagen I and collagen III within the hypertrophic scar.

SPECIAL CONSIDERATIONS IN WOUND HEALING
Traumatic Contaminated Wounds

As discussed previously as a tenet for proper wound healing, wound beds should be optimized through the removal of foreign bodies. This is particularly true for contaminated wounds, and use of pulsed lavage irrigation using several liters of irrigant is ideal.[25] In addition, delayed primary closure is a common technique in the management of contaminated or infected lacerations. This allows a period of dressing changes and wound cleaning that promotes healthy granulation tissue and a decrease of the bacterial burden.

Open Wounds

Secondary healing continues to be a mainstay of treatment in situations where primary closure is not possible. Studies have demonstrated excellent cosmetic outcomes of secondary intention healing when properly applied to specific areas of the face. Evidence suggests that small wounds less than 2 cm in size and located in concave surfaces of the face are ideal conditions for secondary healing **(Table 5)**.[60]

Management of Avulsed Tissue

The literature does not support a definitive treatment for nearly avulsed or avulsed tissue other than to promote microvasculature reanastomosis of avulsed tissue when possible. Although microvasculature reanastomosis is often not an option, reimplantation should be attempted regardless. This rationale stems from the highly vascular nature of the face, which improves the viability of degloved tissues compared with other regions of the body.[55,61] Contraindications to reimplantation include frank necrosis of the avulsed tissue. Because degloving or avulsion injuries are often associated with tissue loss secondary to hypoxia of the reimplanted flap, HBO therapy may facilitate tissue survival.

Future Considerations in Wound Healing

Recent research studying the use of growth factors in optimizing wound healing shows promise. Recombinant human PDGF, becaplermin, was the first Food and Drug Administration–approved growth factor product to treat wounds. Known for

| Table 5 |
| Association between cosmetic outcome and wound size |

	Number of Patients	
Wound Size	Poor/Good Results	Excellent Results
<1 cm	8	9
1–2 cm	18	26
2–3 cm	6	3
3–4 cm	12	3
>4 cm	10	0

Data from van der Eerden PA, Lohuis FJ, Hart AA, et al. Secondary intention healing after excision of nonmelanoma skin cancer of the head and neck: statistical evaluation of prognostic values of wound characteristics and final cosmetic results. Plast Reconstr Surg 2008;122:1747.

increasing soft tissue granulation tissue in diabetic foot ulcers, rhPDGF is also used off-label to induce granulation formation in head and neck wounds.[62] rhPDGF has also been shown to improve the healing of previously irradiated dermal wounds and pharyngocutaneous fistulas.[63,64] As with the clinical use of other growth factors, practitioners should be aware of the theoretic risk of local neoplastic recurrence or malignant transformation.[27]

Autologous platelet-rich plasma, which has been used to reduce bleeding and edema postoperatively, may also improve wound healing. Platelet-rich plasma has been shown to hasten wound closure in full-thickness dermal wounds in healthy individuals.[65] In addition, epidermal growth factor has been shown to enhance the rate of healing of partial-thickness wounds.[27] The use of growth factors prophylactically to improve soft tissue healing has shown promise in both animal and human research.

Prophylactic use of fibroblastic growth factor 1 in the porcine model has decreased radiation injury and reduced adverse postsurgical healing in irradiated skin.[66]

TGF-β continues to be implicated in aberrant healing, and it may be a principal target for future antiscarring therapies. TGF-β expression is altered in keloids and down-regulation of TGF-B1 expression via gene therapy has resulted in decreased scarring in rats.[67,68] Hepatocyte growth factor demonstrates its antifibrotic effects via antagonism of TGF-β.[69] Optimal wound care in the future may involve the use of growth factors more commonly in the management of both acute and chronic wounds.

SUMMARY

The healing of a wound is an intricate process, and the subsequent complications of a wound can be diverse. They can range from acute problems, such as infection, tissue necrosis, dehiscence, and slowed healing, to more chronic complications, such as nonhealing wounds, hypertrophic or atrophic scarring, hyperpitmented or hypopigmented scarring, and keloid formation.

With the exception of keloids (not discussed in this article), most complications improve over time. Study of the different phases of wound healing demonstrates that factors prolonging inflammation can lead to diminished healing and poor cosmesis. Likewise, specific systemic diseases or medications that impede wound healing must be identified, and patients' nutritional status should always be assessed and optimized.

Maintaining a moist environment is imperative for optimal healing, and this can be accomplished by use of topical ointments and semiocclusive or occlusive dressings. Surgical tenets, including aseptic technique, gentle handling of the tissue, strict hemostasis, and avoidance of tension, are key factors in optimal wound healing. Proper selection of cleaning agents, topical medicines, and dressings, to optimize wound healing, continues to be an area of controversy. Through continued research, ways to play a more active and positive role in the wound healing process are being discovered.

REFERENCES

1. Goodman JF, Tanna N, Arden RL, et al. Fundamentals of wound Healing. 3rd edition. San Diego (CA): Pleural Publishing; 2011.

2. Fisher E, Frodel JL. Wound healing. 2nd edition. New York: Thieme; 2002.

3. Saski GH, Krizek TJ. Biology of tissue injury and repair. Baltimore (MD): Williams & Wilkins; 1967.

4. Grinnell F, Billingham RE, Burgess L. Distribution of fibronectin during wound healing in vivo. J Invest Dermatol 1981;76(3):181–9.

5. Leibovich SJ, Ross R. The role of the macrophage in wound repair. A study with hydrocortisone and anti-macrophage serum. Am J Pathol 1975;78(1):71–100.

6. Herndon DN, Nguyen TT, Gilpin DA. Growth factors. Local and systemic. Arch Surg 1993;128(11):1227–33.

7. Howes EL, Sooy JW, Harvey SC. The healing of wounds as determined by their tensile strength. JAMA 1929;92:42.

8. Goslen J. Physiology of wound healing and scar formation. St Louis (MO): CV Mosby; 1989.

9. Winter GD, Scales JT. Effect of air drying and dressings on the surface of a wound. Nature 1963;197:91–2.

10. Hom D. Wound healing in relation to scarring. Facial Plast Surg Clin North Am 1998;6:111.

11. VanWinkle W. The fibroblast in wound healing. Surg Gynecol Obstet 1967;124:369.

12. Stegman SJ, Tromovitch T, Glogau RG. Grafts. Chicago: Year Book Medical Publishers; 1982.

13. Goodson WH 3rd, Hunt TK. Wound healing and aging. J Invest Dermatol 1979;73(1):88–91.

14. Reed BR, Clark RA. Cutaneous tissue repair: practical implications of current knowledge. II. J Am Acad Dermatol 1985;13(6):919–41.

15. Falcone RE, Nappi JF. Chemotherapy and wound healing. Surg Clin North Am 1984;64(4):779–94.

16. Best WR, Khuri SF, Phelan M, et al. Identifying patient preoperative risk factors and postoperative adverse events in administrative databases: results from the Department of Veterans Affairs National Surgical Quality Improvement Program. J Am Coll Surg 2002;194(3):257–66.

17. Franz MG, Steed DL, Robson MC. Optimizing healing of the acute wound by minimizing complications. Curr Probl Surg 2007;44(11):691–763.

18. Brown SA, Coimbra M, Coberly DM, et al. Oral nutritional supplementation accelerates skin wound healing: a randomized, placebo-controlled, double-arm, crossover study. Plast Reconstr Surg 2004;114(1):237–44.

19. Goslen JB. Wound healing for the dermatologic surgeon. J Dermatol Surg Oncol 1988;14(9):959–72.

20. Cooper ML, Laxer JA, Hansbrough JF. The cytotoxic effects of commonly used topical antimicrobial agents on human fibroblasts and keratinocytes. J Trauma 1991;31(6):775–82 [discussion: 782–4].

21. Greenberg L, Ingalls JW. Bactericide/leukocide ratio: a technique for the evaluation of disinfectants. J Am Pharm Assoc Am Pharm Assoc (Baltim) 1958;47(7):531–3.

22. Lineaweaver W, Howard R, Soucy D, et al. Topical antimicrobial toxicity. Arch Surg 1985;120(3):267–70.

23. Drosou A, Falabella A, Kirsner RS. Antiseptics on wounds: an area of controversy. Wounds 2003;15(5). Available at: http://www.medscape.com/viewarticle/456300. Accessed December 25, 2010.

24. Fernandez R, Griffiths R. Water for wound cleansing. Cochrane Database Syst Rev 2008;1:CD003861.

25. Svoboda SJ, Bice TG, Gooden HA, et al. Comparison of bulb syringe and pulsed lavage irrigation with use of a bioluminescent musculoskeletal wound model. J Bone Joint Surg Am 2006;88(10):2167–74.

26. Baranoski S, Ayello E. Wound care essentials practice principles. 2nd edition. Ambler (PA): Williams and Wilkins; 2008.

27. Hom DB, Sun GH, Elluru RG. A contemporary review of wound healing in otolaryngology: current state and future promise. Laryngoscope 2009;119(11):2099–110.

28. Al-Abdullah T, Plint AC, Fergusson D. Absorbable versus nonabsorbable sutures in the management of traumatic lacerations and surgical wounds: a meta-analysis. Pediatr Emerg Care 2007;23(5):339–44.

29. Farion K, Osmond MH, Hartling L, et al. Tissue adhesives for traumatic lacerations in children and adults. Cochrane Database Syst Rev 2002;3:CD003326.

30. Zempsky WT, Parrotti D, Grem C, et al. Randomized controlled comparison of cosmetic outcomes of simple facial lacerations closed with Steri Strip Skin Closures or Dermabond tissue adhesive. Pediatr Emerg Care 2004;20(8):519–24.

31. Chen MA, Davidson TM. Scar management: prevention and treatment strategies. Curr Opin Otolaryngol Head Neck Surg 2005;13(4):242–7.

32. Janis JE, Kwon RK, Lalonde DH. A practical guide to wound healing. Plast Reconstr Surg 2010;125(6):230e–44e.

33. Smack DP, Harrington AC, Dunn C, et al. Infection and allergy incidence in ambulatory surgery patients using white petrolatum vs bacitracin ointment. A randomized controlled trial. JAMA 1996;276(12): 972–7.

34. Fraki JE, Peltonen L, Hopsu-Havu VK. Allergy to various components of topical preparations in stasis dermatitis and leg ulcer. Contact Dermatitis 1979; 5(2):97–100.

35. Atiyeh BS, Amm CA, El Musa KA. Improved scar quality following primary and secondary healing of cutaneous wounds. Aesthetic Plast Surg 2003; 27(5):411–7.

36. Leventhal D, Furr M, Reiter D. Treatment of keloids and hypertrophic scars: a meta-analysis and review of the literature. Arch Facial Plast Surg 2006;8(6): 362–8.

37. Sherris DA, Larrabee WF Jr, Murakami CS. Management of scar contractures, hypertrophic scars, and keloids. Otolaryngol Clin North Am 1995;28(5): 1057–68.

38. McCoy BJ, Diegelmann RF, Cohen IK. In vitro inhibition of cell growth, collagen synthesis, and prolyl hydroxylase activity by triamcinolone acetonide. Proc Soc Exp Biol Med 1980;163(2):216–22.

39. Darzi MA, Chowdri NA, Kaul SK, et al. Evaluation of various methods of treating keloids and hypertrophic scars: a 10-year follow-up study. Br J Plast Surg Jul 1992;45(5):374–9.

40. Ketchum LD, Smith J, Robinson DW, et al. The treatment of hypertrophic scar, keloid and scar contracture by triamcinolone acetonide. Plast Reconstr Surg 1966;38(3):209–18.

41. Saulis AS, Mogford JH, Mustoe TA. Effect of Mederma on hypertrophic scarring in the rabbit ear model. Plast Reconstr Surg 2002;110(1):177–83 [discussion: 184–6].

42. Chung VQ, Kelley L, Marra D, et al. Onion extract gel versus petrolatum emollient on new surgical scars: prospective double-blinded study. Dermatol Surg 2006;32(2):193–7.

43. Chan KY, Lau CL, Adeeb SM, et al. A randomized, placebo-controlled, double-blind, prospective clinical trial of silicone gel in prevention of hypertrophic scar development in median sternotomy wound. Plast Reconstr Surg 2005;116(4):1013–20 [discussion: 1021–12].

44. Bianchi FA, Roccia F, Fiorini P, et al. Use of patient and observer scar assessment scale for evaluation of facial scars treated with self-drying silicone gel. J Craniofac Surg 2010;21(3):719–23.

45. Roseborough IE, Grevious MA, Lee RC. Prevention and treatment of excessive dermal scarring. J Natl Med Assoc 2004;96(1):108–16.

46. Larson DL, Abston S, Willis B, et al. Contracture and scar formation in the burn patient. Clin Plast Surg 1974;1(4):653–6.

47. Richard R, Johnson RM. Managing superficial burn wounds. Adv Skin Wound Care 2002;15(5):246–7.

48. Landau AG, Hudson DA, Adams K, et al. Full-thickness skin grafts: maximizing graft take using negative pressure dressings to prepare the graft bed. Ann Plast Surg 2008;60(6):661–6.

49. DeFranzo AJ, Marks MW, Argenta LC, et al. Vacuum-assisted closure for the treatment of degloving injuries. Plast Reconstr Surg 1999;104(7):2145–8.

50. Blackburn JH 2nd, Boemi L, Hall WW, et al. Negative-pressure dressings as a bolster for skin grafts. Ann Plast Surg 1998;40(5):453–7.

51. Hunt TK, Pai MP. The effect of varying ambient oxygen tensions on wound metabolism and collagen synthesis. Surg Gynecol Obstet 1972;135(4):561–7.

52. Uhl E, Sirsjo A, Haapaniemi T, et al. Hyperbaric oxygen improves wound healing in normal and ischemic skin tissue. Plast Reconstr Surg 1994; 93(4):835–41.

53. Thom SR. Hyperbaric oxygen: its mechanisms and efficacy. Plast Reconstr Surg 2011;127(Suppl 1): 131S–41S.

54. Khandelwal S, Wall J, Kaide C, et al. Case report: successful use of hyperbaric oxygen therapy for a complete scalp degloving injury. Undersea Hyperb Med 2008;35(6):441–5.

55. Cantarella G, Mazzola RF, Pagani D. The fate of an amputated nose after replantation. Am J Otolaryngol 2005;26(5):344–7.

56. Matos LA, Lopez EA, Shellenberger T. Perioperative HBO in head and neck reconstruction with surgical flaps into radiated tissue. 2000. Available at: http://archive.rubicon-foundation.org/4993. Accessed December 25, 2010.

57. Gassner HG, Sherris DA. Chemoimmobilization: improving predictability in the treatment of facial scars. Plast Reconstr Surg 2003;112(5):1464–6.

58. Gassner HG, Brissett AE, Otley CC, et al. Botulinum toxin to improve facial wound healing: a prospective, blinded, placebo-controlled study. Mayo Clin Proc 2006;81(8):1023–8.

59. Wang L, Tai NZ, Fan ZH. [Effect of botulinum toxin type A injection on hypertrophic scar in rabbit ear model]. Zhonghua Zheng Xing Wai Ke Za Zhi Jul 2009;25(4):284–7 [in Chinese].

60. van der Eerden PA, Lohuis PJ, Hart AA, et al. Secondary intention healing after excision of nonmelanoma skin cancer of the head and neck: statistical evaluation of prognostic values of wound characteristics and final cosmetic results. Plast Reconstr Surg 2008;122(6):1747–55.

61. Venter TH, Duminy FJ. Microvascular replantation of avulsed tissue after a dog bite of the face. S Afr Med J 1994;84(1):37–9.

62. Wieman TJ. Clinical efficacy of becaplermin (rhPDGF-BB) gel. Becaplermin Gel Studies Group. Am J Surg 1998;176(2A Suppl):74S–9S.

63. Hom DB, Manivel JC. Promoting healing with recombinant human platelet-derived growth factor–BB in a previously irradiated problem wound. Laryngoscope 2003;113(9):1566–71.

64. Jakubowicz DM, Smith RV. Use of becaplermin in the closure of pharyngocutaneous fistulas. Head Neck 2005;27(5):433–8.

65. Hom DB, Linzie BM, Huang TC. The healing effects of autologous platelet gel on acute human skin wounds. Arch Facial Plast Surg 2007;9(3): 174–83.

66. Hom DB, Unger GM, Pernell KJ, et al. Improving surgical wound healing with basic fibroblast growth factor after radiation. Laryngoscope 2005;115(3): 412–22.

67. Xia W, Phan TT, Lim IJ, et al. Complex epithelial-mesenchymal interactions modulate transforming growth factor-beta expression in keloid-derived cells. Wound Repair Regen 2004;12(5):546–56.

68. Liu W, Wang DR, Cao YL. TGF-beta: a fibrotic factor in wound scarring and a potential target for anti-scarring gene therapy. Curr Gene Ther 2004;4(1):123–36.

69. Ono I, Yamashita T, Hida T, et al. Local administration of hepatocyte growth factor gene enhances the regeneration of dermis in acute incisional wounds. J Surg Res 2004;120(1):47–55.

Keloids: Prevention and Management

Douglas M. Sidle, MD[a],*, Haena Kim, MD[b]

KEYWORDS

- Keloid • Scar management • Hypertrophic scars
- Wound healing • Keloid pathophysiology

Key Points

- Keloids can be difficult to differentiate clinically from hypertrophic scars; however, there are distinguishing characteristics of each
- The pathophysiology of keloids continues to require ongoing research
- Surgical excision followed by intralesional steroid injection is considered a first line treatment
- Silastic gel sheeting can improve keloid appearance when used appropriately
- Radiation can be a safe and effective means of keloid treatment with the appropriate precautions
- Topical application of chemotherapy medication is a reasonable alternative in patients with keloid recurrence after surgical excision and steroid treatment

---

PATHOPHYSIOLOGY AND HISTOLOGY

Wound healing is tightly regulated, and errors in the process can manifest anywhere along the pathologic spectrum from chronic wounds to the aggressive scar formation seen in keloids, the latter being the topic of interest here. On the subject of keloids, hypertrophic scars must also be mentioned because the two are often, incorrectly, used interchangeably. This distinction must be made, as the appropriate application of current and future interventions mandates understanding the clinical, histologic, and biochemical pathology of keloids.

Keloids can occur immediately after trauma, or grow months after a mature, stable scar has formed. This trauma can range from vaccination needle sticks, lacerations, bug bites, and burns, to dermatologic conditions such as acne or folliculitis. In all cases, the end result is skin inflammation. Hypertrophic scars follow the pattern of evolution, stabilization, and involution within the boundaries of the original wound. By contrast, keloids continue to proliferate, resulting in a raised, erythematous scar with a wide variability of height progression and scar distribution. As such, keloids will grow outside the boundaries of the original scar. Although keloids can reach a quiescent phase, very rarely do they regress. Lee and colleagues[1] found that symptomatically, 46% of patients noted keloid-associated pain and 86% noted pruritis.[2]

Keloids affect darker-skinned individuals approximately 15 times more than Caucasians, suggesting a genetic factor. Keloids affect roughly 15% to 20% of the African American and Hispanic populations.[3,4] Keloids typically occur during and after puberty, between the ages of 10 and 30 years. Although there is no gender predilection, keloids can regress during menopause or worsen during pregnancy.

Disclosure Statement: The authors have no financial obligations to disclose.
[a] Division of Facial Plastic Surgery, Department of Otolaryngology–Head and Neck Surgery, Northwestern University Feinberg School of Medicine, 676 North Street Clair, Suite 1325, Chicago, IL 60611, USA
[b] Department of Otolaryngology–Head and Neck Surgery, McGaw Medical Center, Northwestern University Feinberg School of Medicine, 676 North Street Clair, Suite 1325, Chicago, IL 60611, USA
* Corresponding author.
E-mail address: drsidle@yahoo.com

Facial Plast Surg Clin N Am 19 (2011) 505–515
doi:10.1016/j.fsc.2011.06.005
1064-7406/11/$ – see front matter © 2011 Elsevier Inc. All rights reserved.

The pathogenesis of keloids continues to undergo investigation, and understanding this process requires knowledge of the normal wound-healing process. Normal wound healing occurs in 3 stages[3]: the inflammatory phase,[4] the proliferative/granulation phase, and[5] the maturation/remodeling phase. The inflammatory phase begins immediately after the injury. Hemostatic mechanisms of platelet degranulation and activation of complement and clotting cascades occur quickly. Cytokines and growth factors such as transforming growth factor β (TGF-β), platelet derived growth factor (PDGF), and epidermal growth factor (EGF) are released through platelet degranulation and from the surrounding tissue.[6,7] These cytokines and growth factors induce the influx of neutrophils, macrophages, mast cells, and epithelial cells.[6] After the first 24 to 48 hours, the inflammation is perpetuated by mast cells and neutrophils and can last for anywhere from 3 to 8 days.[3,8] Macrophages aid in wound debridement as fibroblasts and smooth muscle cells migrate into the wound. Prolongation of this phase occurs in cases of large wounds or in the presence of infection, and results in greater exposure to fibrogenic cytokines.[6]

During the proliferative phase, at approximately 3 to 6 weeks, fibroblasts deposit type III collagen and synthesize granulation tissue, composed of procollagen, elastin, proteoglycans, and hyaluronic acid.[8] This scaffold allows the ingrowth of vasculature, and with wound contracture and closure facilitated by myofibroblasts, allows the wound to undergo continued remodeling in the final phase of wound healing.

The maturation/remodeling phase can take from several months to more than a year. During this phase, the type III collagen is replaced by stronger type I collagen fibers. Proteoglycans are synthesized, and fibrin and fibronectin are degraded. In addition, the extracellular matrix produced by fibroblasts undergoes simultaneous degradation by mostly serine proteases (ie, tissue plasminogen activator and urokinase plasminogen activator) and matrix metalloproteinases (MMPs). Collagen fibers are rearranged, cross-linked, and aligned along tension lines. The tensile strength of the scar improves, but at best achieves only 80% the tensile strength of normal skin.[3]

Histologically, keloids invade the normal surrounding dermis, a distinct difference from hypertrophic scars, which stay within the confines of the wound borders. In keloids, collagen fibers are larger, thicker, wavier, and oriented haphazardly. Collagen fibers in hypertrophic scars and normal scars are oriented parallel to the epidermal surface.[9] The collagen fibers in keloids are arranged into thick collagen bundles that are packed tightly together within the dermis, where there is a lack of sebaceous glands and rete ridges.[10,11] These collagen bundles are also found to lack the presence of myofibroblasts. Hypertrophic scars form fibrous nodules composed of fibroblasts, mostly type III collagen fibers, and vessels.[8,12] By contrast, keloid scars form nodules with reduced vascularity and a hypocellular appearance (Fig. 1).[4,8,12,13] This acellular core within keloids is characterized by thick bundles of type I and type III collagen fibers interspersed with fibroblasts (see Fig. 1B).[8,12,13]

Summarizing the overall histologic findings of keloids, Butler and colleagues[4] classified 4 distinct pathognomonic findings on histology:

1. Keloidal hyalinized collagen
2. Tongue-like advancing edge underneath normal-appearing epidermis and papillary dermis
3. Horizontal cellular fibrous bands in upper reticular dermis
4. Prominent fascia-like fibrous bands.

Despite advances in histologic knowledge of keloids, their exact pathogenesis and etiology remain unclear. Accordingly, the number of possible treatment options reflects multiple hypotheses on how the normal wound-healing process goes awry in keloids. The authors review here the most common theories that are based on accepted observations and proposed contributing factors.

Growth Factors

Elevated levels of TGF-β and PDGF have been found in keloid tissue along with aberrant levels of their activity. The heightened growth-factor activity is likely a result of increased expression of their respective receptors.[3,14,15] TGF-β stimulates fibroblasts to produce and deposit collagen and extracellular matrix (ECM) factors. Of interest, keloid fibroblasts exhibit a heightened sensitivity to this growth factor. TGF-β also induces production of PDGF, which controls the rate of granulation tissue formation and stimulates collagen production during the later stages of wound healing.[3] Furthermore, the enzymes that remodel and break down scar ECM are regulated by TGF-β, and decreased levels of collagenase, plasminogen activator, and MMPs could further explain the failure of scar regression evidenced in keloids.

Genetics

Keloids occur more commonly in those of African, Asian, and Hispanic descent, suggesting a genetic susceptibility in darker-skinned individuals. Familial cases of an autosomal dominant pattern of keloids have been reported, and further genetic

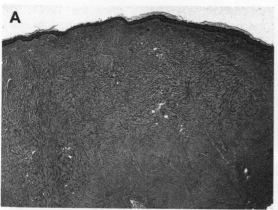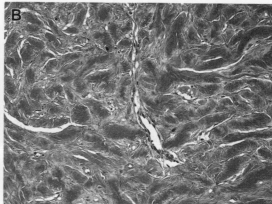

Fig. 1. Keloid histopathology on low power (*A*) and high power (*B*). Abundant collagen fibers contribute to the nodular appearance of the dermis (*A*). Higher power view of keloid scar highlights hyalinized collagen fibers interspersed with fibroblasts with linearized blood vessels (*B*). Also, note the lack of epidermal appendages on both low and high power (*A*, hematoxylin-eosin, original magnification ×20; *B*, H&E, original magnification ×200). (*Courtesy of* Pedram Pouryazdanparast, MD.)

studies have linked keloid occurrence to loci on chromosomes 2 and 7.[3,9,16,17] Variable gene expression and polygenetic inheritance pattern makes identification of a single gene difficult.[3,16] In the general population, however, no single gene is responsible for keloid formation.[3]

Dysregulation of apoptosis and altered tumor suppressor gene expression have also been proposed mechanisms of pathogenesis, and studies on p53 and Stat-3 have shown elevated levels compared with normal fibroblasts.[18,19] Various HLA types have been found to correlate with the keloid phenotype in a Caucasian and Chinese Han population: HLA-DR5, HLA-DQ23, HLA-DQA1, and HLA-DQB1.[3,20–23] This finding suggests an abnormal immune response to skin injury in the form of a local immune reaction or possibly a cell-mediated autoimmune reaction.[3]

Skin Trauma

Keloids typically occur after an inciting event, and scar contracture is a necessary step in normal wound healing. Excess mechanical strain on a wound outside of relaxed skin tension lines is a proposed mechanism of keloid formation.[3–5] Keloids typically occur in younger individuals, a population that naturally possesses greater skin elasticity and tensile strength; this could translate into greater wound tension, mechanical strain, and further influx of hyperfunctioning fibroblasts. Others, however, debate this theory, as some of the most common areas of occurrence are under the least tension (ie, ear, back of the neck).[3,5] Conversely, the palms and soles of the feet, areas under high tension, are rarely affected.[3,5]

Given the multitude of contributing factors to the pathophysiology of keloids, treatment options are abundant. Despite numerous options, many investigators agree that the most efficacious route is prevention of keloid formation. In those individuals with a predilection to formation of keloids, caution must be exercised with any procedure that can lead to skin inflammation. Care must be taken to reduce skin tension, wound infection, and foreign-body reaction, with formalized treatment reserved for true keloids and not immature scars.

TREATMENT OPTIONS
Steroids

Injection of corticosteroids is frequently employed as first-line therapy for keloids. Although steroids can be used as monotherapy, optimal results have been reported with its use as adjuvant or combination treatment (ie, surgery, cryotherapy, pulse-dye laser, and 5-fluorouracil [5-FU][24–27]). Successful application of steroid injections requires injection into the scar itself, which can be a painful procedure for the patient. Steroids have been shown to induce keloid regression by decreasing collagen and glycosaminoglycan synthesis, reducing the inflammatory process and fibroblast proliferation, and inducing tissue hypoxia through vasoconstriction. In addition, corticosteroids have been found to result in decreased levels of TGF-β and decreased angiogenesis by suppressing endogenous vascular EGF.[28,29] Side effects can include skin atrophy, depigmentation, telangiectasias, atrophy of subcutaneous tissue and fat, skin necrosis, ulcerations, and Cushingoid features.

Steroid injections as monotherapy have variable efficacy rates ranging from 50% to 100% and recurrence rates from 9% to 50%.[24,25] Higher success rates can be achieved when treating young, proliferative scars. Several alternative steroid preparations can be employed: hydrocortisone acetate, methylprednisolone acetate, dexamethasone, and triamcinolone acetonide (TA). Although TA is the most frequently employed, there appears to be no benefit derived from using one steroid over another. Numerous therapeutic regimens have been published that commonly tailor dosage and number of treatments based on keloid size and site of the scar. Recommendations vary, from starting dosages of 10 mg/mL to 40 mg/mL of triamcinolone. In the literature, as much as 80 to 120 mg/mL has been used for larger keloids.[5,30] However, the unifying theme of treatment plans for larger keloids involves frequent scheduled sessions, typically on a monthly basis, for 2 to 3 dosages and may require sporadic treatment for up to 6 months.[24,25,28] Because of the pain associated with intralesional injection, many physicians opt to pretreat with lidocaine. The authors prefer to add 1% lidocaine in equal volume to the steroid dose.

With regard to the pediatric population, a great degree of caution must be employed when using corticosteroids. Treatment of children should be monitored closely and have a regularly scheduled follow-up. Various regimens combining TA with other modalities such as 5-FU or pulsed dye laser have been evaluated.[31,32] Manuskiatti and Fitzpatrick[31] did not find a significant difference in treatment outcome when comparing combination therapy with TA alone. However, these investigators did find faster improvement in keloid appearance using intralesional TA, 5-FU, or both when compared with pulsed dye laser alone. By contrast, Asilian and colleagues[32] showed improved results when combining triamcinolone, 5-FU, and pulsed dye laser.

Despite conflicting data, combination therapy can be a reasonable option in patients who do not respond to single-modality treatment. Nevertheless, TA alone does remain a widely accepted first-line treatment. The publication of international guidelines for scar management in 2002 has further solidified the role of intralesional steroids in the treatment of keloids.[33] This panel further proposed that optimal outcomes are achieved when combining surgical excision and intradermal delivery of corticosteroids.[33]

Compression

Compression therapy has been employed since the 1840s and has been commonly used for prophylaxis after burns since the 1970s. The mechanism of its action has yet to be fully elucidated. However, there are multiple theories[8,34]:

1. A decrease in blood flow with a resultant decrease in α2-macroglobulin and increase in collagenase-mediated collagen breakdown, normally inhibited by α2-macroglobulin
2. Hypoxia leading to fibroblast degeneration and collagen degradation
3. Lower levels of chondroitin-4-sulfate with increase in collagen degradation
4. Decreased scar hydration, resulting in mast cell stabilization and decrease in neovascularization and matrix production.

Another more recently proposed theory suggests that tissue remodeling is induced by the stimulation of mechanoreceptors. Mechanoreceptors have been found to contribute to cellular apoptosis and overall tissue remodeling by increasing the rigidity of scar extracellular matrix and discouraging the differentiation and proliferation of fibroblasts.[35]

Compression therapy can be difficult for patients to tolerate, as it requires patient adherence to a strict regimen. The goal of compression therapy is to exceed the inherent capillary pressure of 24 mm Hg. Described treatments require the use of compression garments or devices day and night for 6 to 12 months with discontinuation of pressure kept to less than 30 minutes per day.[34] There is a wide variety of commercial materials available for use. A few examples include Coban bandages (3M, St Paul, MN), support bandages and presized garments (Jobst, Toledo, OH), and pressure earrings. While compression therapy has been found to be beneficial, patient compliance can be the limiting factor due to duration of treatment.[34]

Although the use of silicone gel sheeting does not produce much true compression, some investigators do include it in the category of compression therapy. The use of silicone gel sheeting (SGS) is one of the few treatment modalities for keloids that have undergone evaluation in controlled trials. SGS has been found to be highly effective as a prophylactic measure in high-risk individuals, and improves overall scar appearance (ie, elevation, elasticity, redness, and so forth).[24,25] Other modalities of silicone application include cream containing 20% silicone oil followed by an occlusive dressing that is air-permeable but water-impermeable. More commonly used is a self-drying topical silicone gel that dries to form a flexible, occlusive dressing of silicone, such as Scarguard MD® (Scarguard Labs, Great Neck, NY, USA). Scarguard MD® is a quick-drying liquid containing silicone (12.75%), hydrocortisone (0.55%), and vitamin E, and its use is initiated typically 2 weeks after surgery. Comparative controlled studies have shown that silicone gel is equally as effective as SGS in treating keloids and abnormal scarring.[24,36–38] Furthermore, it has been rated by patients as easier to use than SGS.[24]

The efficacy of silicone-based products is likely not attributable to altered oxygen tension, blood flow, or the entry of silicone in scar tissue.[24,25,39] One theory suggests altered kinetics of collagenase and resulting scar formation due to an increase in skin surface temperature of approximately 1.7°C (approximately 35°F) while using SGS.[40–42] One group has proposed that SGS reduces tension at the borders of keloid scars.[33] Another popular theory is that SGS increases tissue hydration by decreasing water evaporation in the stratum corneum. This theory is based on the observation that full-thickness wounds result in injury to the stratum corneum and disruption of the normal fluid homeostasis of the epithelium. The resulting transepidermal water loss can take a year to normalize, and has been found to be higher in cases of excessive scarring when compared with normal skin. This process could lead to increased stimulation of fibroblast collagen production and deposition. Both SGS and silicone gel/cream therapies with occlusive dressing likely restore the epithelial fluid homeostasis to similar degrees.[24,25,41] The restoration of the balance of hydration/rehydration by SGS and silicone gel is unique, as similar scar effects have not been found with an occlusive dressing alone.[24]

Surgery

Surgical treatment of keloids can be employed to either reduce keloid mass or radically remove the keloid. **Fig. 2** is an example of a left pinna keloid in a 25-year-old Caucasian woman. This patient formed a keloid secondary to ear piercing, and she is currently without recurrence after excision and steroid injections. The reduction of keloid mass without complete extirpation can be used in cases of infection or alleviation of symptoms secondary to keloid mass. Complete excision of keloids is associated with high recurrence rates (50%–100%), and should usually be combined with adjuvant therapies.

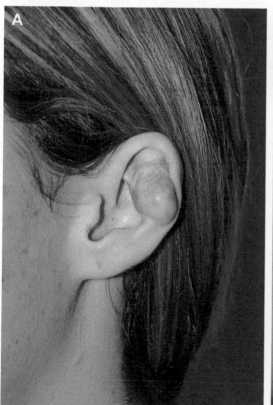 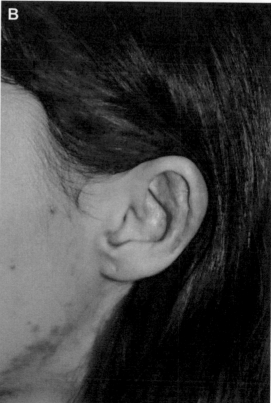

Fig. 2. Caucasian patient pretreatment (*A*) and 6 months postexcision (*B*) of helix keloid. The patient underwent subcutaneous excision of keloid, primary closure, and adjuvant corticosteroid injection. The patient is still without recurrence.

The surgeon has the option of anesthetizing the site with a combination of equal parts triamcinolone (40 mg/mL) with lidocaine with epinephrine.[43,44] If the lesion is pedunculated, an elliptical excision should be performed, followed by undermining of the surrounding skin before closure with sutures. For broader-based sessile lesions, one investigator recommends an alternative closure. Kelly[43] recommends a U-shaped incision when excising large sessile keloids. This U-shaped incision produces a tongue-like flap of keloid tissue. Kelly plans the skin flap to be one-fifth the size of the keloid from its border to the flattest-looking surface. The keloid is excised followed by closure of the site with the tongue-like flap of keloid tissue. Also recommended is suture removal after 10 to 20 days, especially in the case of earlobe keloids.[43]

When operating on a patient with a known history of keloids, care must be taken to follow relaxed skin tension lines. Closure of the defect should be done with maximal wound edge eversion, and minimum tension.[5,43] Mustoe advocates splinting of the tissue with permanent intradermal sutures (clear nylon), and subcuticular closure with nonabsorbable polypropylene sutures to be left in place for 6 months. However the author does not specify if sutures should be removed or left in situ. Mustoe[25] believes absorbable sutures lose tensile strength too quickly (<1 month) to effectively splint the wound to prevent scar widening or scar hypertrophy. He uses hypoallergenic microporous tape to minimize wound shearing followed by application of SGS as prophylaxis. Mustoe encourages that SGS should be worn for a minimum of 12 hours a day for up to 1 month.

Radiation

Radiation has been used for treatment of keloids since the late 1800s, and there are multiple radiation protocols for keloid treatment, which vary in the type of beam used and the use of radiation as monotherapy or adjuvant therapy. The most common use of radiation is as adjuvant postoperative treatment, although this has not been evaluated in a randomized, prospective controlled trial. Success rates have been recorded in the range of 67% to 98%.[26,27] Of course there remains some trepidation among physicians regarding the use of radiation to treat a benign disease. Many physicians fear that the use of radiation could produce malignant transformation. In 2009 Ogawa and colleagues[26] conducted a literature search evaluating radiation-associated carcinogenesis between the years 1901 and 2009, and found only 5 reported cases, one of which was a likely malignant

transformation of keloid.[26] In the remaining 4 cases the radiation doses and documentation of appropriate protection of surrounding tissue was inconsistent. Leer and colleagues[45] conducted an international survey of radiation oncologists on the safety of radiation on a range of benign diseases, including keloids. Of the 70 institutions in the United States and Canada, more than 90% believed that radiation is a suitable treatment for keloids.[45] In 2007, Leer and colleagues[46] evaluated the use of radiation in the treatment of benign disease throughout the body and classified its use as category A, an accepted indication. Categories B and C were also established, the former recommending use only in clinical trials and the latter not accepted. When using radiation, appropriate protection of thyroid and breast tissue is essential, and its use should be restricted to adults.

The dosage of radiation can be varied. As such, a balance between safety and efficacy should be sought. Recommended dosages range from 10 to 20 Gy with timing of administration within 2 days after surgery. Doses are tailored for the anatomic site, with higher dosages reserved for sites exposed to greater skin tension (ie, chest wall, shoulder, scapula). In 2007 Ogawa and colleagues[27] recommended radiation protocols depending on anatomic site: (1) anterior chest wall, shoulder-scapular region, suprapubic region, 20 Gy in 4 fractions over 4 days; (2) ear lobe, 10 Gy in 2 fractions over 2 days; and (3) for other sites, 15 Gy in 3 fractions over 3 days. **Fig. 3** is an example of a radiation mask used during treatment sessions. These masks are used to immobilize the patient, with an area cut out over the target. At the authors' institution, immobilization masks are used less frequently. Instead, wires are used to isolate the area to be treated and to form a radiation shield that is shaped to the demarcated area (**Figs. 4** and **5**).

Side effects of radiation can be divided into acute/subacute and late, the former occurring within the first 7 to 10 days and the latter occurring several weeks after exposure. Acute and subacute reactions include erythema, hyperpigmentation, epilation, and desquamation. Later complications range from scarring, permanent pigmentation/depigmentation, and atrophy, to dermal fibrosis and ulceration. Of note, there have been no reports of ulceration or wound dehiscence in the setting of postoperative radiation.[26] **Fig. 6**A and B show a recurrent keloid after surgical excision and numerous treatments with intralesional steroid injections. This patient had recurrence after surgery and steroid treatment (**Fig. 6**C), but good results were finally obtained after excision and postoperative treatment with radiation (**Fig. 6**D).

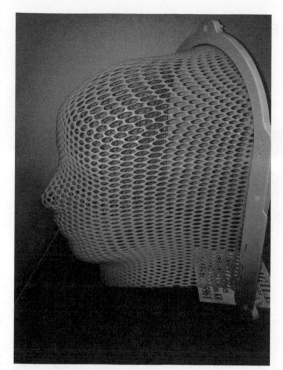

Fig. 3. Radiation mask used during radiation treatment for immobilization.

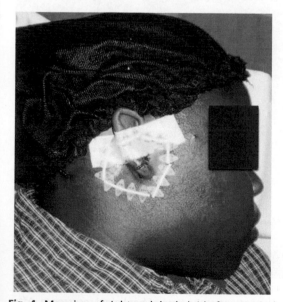

Fig. 4. Mapping of right earlobe keloid after surgical resection for radiation field. Area of interest is encompassed by radiopaque wires. These wires aid in production of a customized shield that protects surrounding tissue during treatment sessions. (*Courtesy of* Haider Shirazi, MD.)

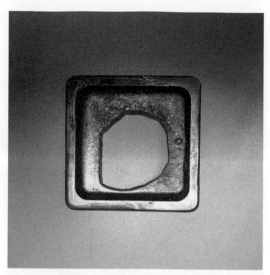

Fig. 5. Example of radiation shield with cut-out customized to the area demarcated by wires. The shield is placed between the patient and the radiation beam source, preventing exposure of surrounding tissue to radiation.

Chemotherapy

The use of antineoplastic agents has emerged as another potential tool for keloid treatment. While efficacy rates and lesion recurrence rates vary from one agent to another, the use of these novel agents, as either monotherapy or adjuvant therapy, continues to undergo investigation. Studies on interferon-α2b (IFN-α2b) and interferon-γ (IFN-γ) have yielded mixed results. In vitro studies have revealed decreased collagen production in keloid tissue after exposure to IFN.[47] Clinical results are varied, with early decreases in keloid size but late recurrences when using IFN-γ. Similarly, no significant decrease in recurrence rates was observed when using IFN-α2b.[48–50]

Bleomycin is a metabolic derivative produced by a strain of *Streptomyces*. It demonstrates antitumor, antiviral, and antibacterial activity, and causes breakage of both single-stranded and double-stranded DNA. Bleomycin's efficacy has been found to be more promising than that of the IFNs. Studies have shown that bleomycin can produce significantly greater regression of larger keloids compared with triamcinolone.[51,52] Aggarwal and colleagues[51] demonstrated encouraging results, with complete flattening of the keloid in 44% to 73% of patients and adequate/significant flattening in another 14% to 22%. Moreover, pruritus was relieved in 89% of their patients. Although systemic side effects can include pulmonary fibrosis or hepatotoxicity, the dosages used for keloid treatment do not approach an amount that would cause these side effects. Shridharani

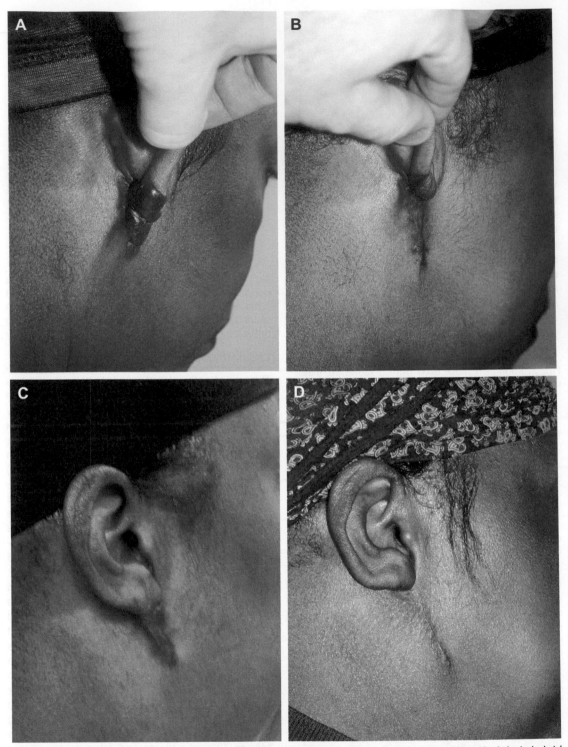

Fig. 6. African American patient with lobule keloid treated initially with surgical excision. (*A*) Right lobule keloid. (*B*) The same patient after her initial surgical resection. (*C*) The patient at the time of her keloid recurrence. After the recurrence, she was treated more aggressively with excision and radiation. Her radiation treatment schedule was 7 fractions at 21 Gy each. (*D*) At 6 months' follow-up the patient is still without recurrence.

and colleagues[50] proposed dosages using a concentration of bleomycin of 1.5 IU/mL, with at most 6 mL used per session. Side effects were local and were restricted to hyperpigmentation and dermal atrophy.

Though limited in subject numbers, studies on the use of mitomycin C have shown interesting results as well. Mitomycin C is an antineoplastic agent that inhibits DNA synthesis by cross-linking DNA strands, thus preventing proliferation. Mitomycin C is frequently used in ophthalmology to prevent scar formation after glaucoma surgery. When applied topically it effectively inhibits fibroblast proliferation at the extraocular drainage site. Reported side effects of topical mitomycin C are minimal, and when mentioned in the literature are limited to hyperpigmentation and skin atrophy.[50,53] Clinical studies have evaluated the use of topical application of mitomycin C after resection of keloids. Although the results are variable, they are encouraging. Stewart and Kim[53] were able to prevent keloid recurrence in 9 of 10 patients up to an average of 8 months postprocedure. This group applied cotton pledgets soaked in mitomycin C (4 mg/5 mL) to the wound bed after keloid excision.[53] Bailey and colleagues[54] had dermatologists, patients, and clinical staff evaluate pretreatment and posttreatment photographs. Although only 10 patients were included in the study, results were graded as satisfactory in 80% of cases.

5-FU, a pyrimidine analogue, has also shown promise in the treatment of keloids. 5-FU can be used either as an Intralesional injection or, less frequently, as a topical soak after surgical excision. The likely mechanism of 5-FU's action is inhibition of TGF-β activation of type I collagen expression in fibroblasts.[55] Clinical results thus far are promising. When studied as monotherapy on keloids younger than 2 years, 5-FU produced complete resolution with no evidence of recurrence at 1 year follow-up in approximately 82%.[56] Kontochristopoulos and colleagues[56] were able to decrease keloid volume in 95% of patients with 5-FU (50 mg/mL) injected over 7 sessions with an average delivered volume of 0.2 to 0.4 mL/cm^2 per spot. Postsurgical topical application of 5-FU to the new scar also produced impressive reduction of recurrence. Only 19% recurred in one study.[57–59] Of interest, all of the patients in the study by Haurani and colleagues[57] had failed prior attempts with intralesional steroid injection.

In conclusion, keloid management remains a frustrating disease for both physician and patient. Successful management requires pretreatment education and counseling, as the recurrence rates are high and some treatment plans are rigorous.

The discussion with the patient should emphasize the importance of treatment compliance in achieving a satisfactory outcome. The topic of keloid recurrence should certainly also be broached at this time. Patient goals should be clearly ascertained. Although the majority of patients' concerns center on aesthetic outcome, there are patients who may simply seek relief from keloid symptoms (ie, pruritus and pain).

Although surgical excision followed by intralesional steroid injection is considered the standard of care, recurrence continues to plague many patients. In some of these select patients, the treating physician may consider alternatives such as topical application of chemotherapeutic agents and radiation. In the case of radiation treatment, a multidisciplinary approach is mandatory, involving the radiation oncologist and the surgeon. The timing of keloid excision with radiation treatment requires coordination and communication between the two departments. Our understanding of keloids and their treatment continues to grow. Although certain options may seem "radical" to patients and physicians alike, it is our responsibility to employ treatments based on the most current medical knowledge. Likewise, as we continue to use newer treatments we must persist in finding the optimal one.

REFERENCES

1. Lee SS, Yosipovitch G, Chan YH. Pruritus, pain, and small nerve fiber function in keloids: a controlled study. J Am Acad Dermatol 2004;51:1002–6.
2. Ogawa R. The most current algorithms for the treatment and prevention of hypertrophic scars and keloids. Plast Reconstr Surg 2010;125(2):557–68.
3. Bran GM, Goessler UR, Hormann K, et al. Keloids: current concepts of pathogenesis (review). Int J Mol Med 2009;24(3):283–93.
4. Butler PD, Longaker MT, Yang GP. Current progress in keloid research and treatment. J Am Coll Surg 2008;206(4):731–41.
5. Robles DT, Moore E, Draznin M, et al. Keloids: pathophysiology and management. Dermatol Online J 2007;13(3):9.
6. Tredget EE, Nedelec B, Scott PG, et al. Hypertrophic scars, keloids, and contractures. The cellular and molecular basis for therapy. Surg Clin North Am 1997;77(3):701–30.
7. Rockwell WB, Cohen IK, Ehrlich HP. Keloids and hypertrophic scars: a comprehensive review. Plast Reconstr Surg 1989;84(5):827–37.
8. Wolfram D, Tzankov A, Pulzl P, et al. Hypertrophic scars and keloids—a review of their pathophysiology, risk factors, and therapeutic management. Dermatol Surg 2009;35(2):171–81.

9. Chike-Obi CJ, Cole PD, Brissett AE. Keloids: pathogenesis, clinical features, and management. Semin Plast Surg 2009;23(3):178–84.

10. Kose O, Waseem A. Keloids and hypertrophic scars: are they two different sides of the same coin? Dermatol Surg 2008;34(3):336–46.

11. Tsao SS, Dover JS, Arndt KA, et al. Scar management: keloid, hypertrophic, atrophic, acne scars. Semin Cutan Med Surg 2002;21(1):46–75.

12. Elder DE, editor. Lever's histopathology of the skin. Philadelphia: Ovid Technologies (online library); 2004.

13. Elder DE, editor. Atlas and synopsis of Lever's histopathology of the skin. Philadelphia: Ovid Technologies (online library); 2007.

14. Al-Attar A, Mess S, Thomassen JM, et al. Keloid pathogenesis and treatment. Plast Reconstr Surg 2006;117(1):286–300.

15. Kelly AP. Medical and surgical therapies for keloids. Dermatol Ther 2004;17(2):212–8.

16. Marneros AG, Norris JE, Olsen BR, et al. Clinical genetics of familial keloids. Arch Dermatol 2001;137:1429–34.

17. Satish L, Lyons-Weiler J, Hebda PA, et al. Gene expression patterns in isolated keloid fibroblasts. Wound Repair Regen 2006;14:463–70.

18. Tanaka A, Hatoko M, Tada H, et al. Expression of p53 family in scars. J Dermatol Sci 2004;34(1):17–24.

19. Lim CP, Phan TT, Lim IJ, et al. Stat3 contributes to keloid pathogenesis via promoting collagen production, cell proliferation and migration. Oncogene 2006; 25:5416–25.

20. Brown JJ, Ollier WE, Thomson W, et al. Positive association of HLA-DRB1*15 with keloid disease in Caucasians. Int J Immunogenet 2008;35(4–5):303–7.

21. Lu WS, Wang JF, Yang S. Association of HLA-DQA1 and DQB1 alleles with keloids in Chinese Hans. J Dermatol Sci 2008;52(2):108–17.

22. Shih B, Bayat A. Genetics of keloid scarring. Arch Dermatol Res 2010;302(5):319–49.

23. Froelich K, Staudenmaier R, Kleinsasser N, et al. Therapy of auricular keloids: review of different treatment modalities and proposal for a therapeutic algorithm. Eur Arch Otorhinolaryngol 2007;264(12):1297–508.

24. Mustoe TA. Evolution of silicone therapy and mechanism of action in scar management. Aesthetic Plast Surg 2008;32(1):82–92.

25. Mustoe TA. Scars and keloids. BMJ 2004;328(7432):1329–30.

26. Ogawa R, Yoshitatsu S, Yoshida K, et al. Is radiation therapy for keloids acceptable? The risk of radiation-induced carcinogenesis. Plast Reconstr Surg 2009; 124(4):1196–201.

27. Ogawa R, Miyashita T, Hyakusoku H, et al. Postoperative radiation protocol for keloids and hypertrophic scars: statistical analysis of 370 sites followed for over 18 months. Ann Plast Surg 2007;59:688–91.

28. Roques C, Teot L. The use of corticosteroids to treat keloids: a review. Int J Low Extrem Wounds 2008; 7(3):137–45.

29. Mustoe TA, Cooter RD, Gold MH, et al. International clinical recommendations on scar management. Plast Reconstr Surg 2002;110(2):560–71.

30. Darzi MA, Chowdri NA, Kaul SK, et al. Evaluation of various methods of treating keloids and hypertrophic scars: a 10-year follow-up study. Br J Plast Surg 1992;45(5):374–9.

31. Manuskiatti W, Fitzpatrick RE. Treatment response of keloidal and hypertrophic sternotomy scars: comparison among intralesional corticosteroid, 5-fluorouracil, and 585-nm flashlamp-pumped pulsed-dye laser treatments. Arch Dermatol 2002;128(9):1149–55.

32. Asilian A, Darouheh A, Shariati F. New combination of triamcinolone, 5-fluorouracil, and pulsed-dye laser for treatment of keloid and hypertrophic scars. Dermatol Surg 2006;32:907–15.

33. Akaishi S, Akimoto M, Hyakusoku H, et al. The tensile reduction effects of silicone gel sheeting. Plast Reconstr Surg 2010;126(2):109e–11e.

34. Urioste SS, Arndt KA, Dover JS. Keloids and hypertrophic scars: review and treatment strategies. Semin Cutan Med Surg 1999;18(2):159–71.

35. Yagmur C, Akaishi S, Ogawa R, et al. Mechanical receptor-related mechanisms in scar management: a review and hypothesis. Plast Reconstr Surg 2010;120(2):426–34.

36. Chan KY, Lau CL, Adeeb SM, et al. A randomized, placebo-controlled, double-blind, prospective clinical trial of silicone gel in prevention of hypertrophic scar development in median sternotomy wound. Plast Reconstr Surg 2005;116:1013–20.

37. Chernoff WG, Cramer H, Su-Huang S. The efficacy of topical silicone gel elastomers in the treatment of hypertrophic scars, keloid scars, and post laser exfoliation erythema. Aesthetic Plast Surg 2007;32(5):495–500.

38. Signorini M, Clementoni MT. Clinical evaluation of a new self-drying silicone gel in the treatment of scars: a preliminary report. Aesthetic Plast Surg 2007; 31(2):183–7.

39. Musgrave MA, Umraw N, Fish JS, et al. The effect of silicone gel sheets on perfusion of hypertrophic burn scars. J Burn Care Rehabil 2002;23:208–14.

40. Borgognoni L. Biological effects of silicone gel sheeting. Wound Repair Regen 2002;10(2):118–21.

41. Lyle WG. Silicone gel sheeting. Plast Reconstr Surg 2001;107(1):272–5.

42. Niessen FB, Spauwen PH, Schalkwijk J, et al. On the nature of hypertrophic scars and keloids: a review. Plast Reconstr Surg 1999;104(5):1435–58.

43. Kelly AP. Update on the management of keloids. Semin Cutan Med Surg 2009;28(2):71–6.

44. Poochareon VN, Berman B. New therapies for the management of keloids. J Craniofac Surg 2003; 14(5):654–7.

45. Leer JW, van Houtte P, Develaar J. Indications and treatment schedules for irradiation of benign disease: a survey. Radiother Oncol 1998;48:249–57.

46. Leer JW, van Houtte P, Seegenschmiedt H. Radiotherapy of non-malignant disorders: where do we stand? Radiother Oncol 2007;83:175–7.

47. Berman B, Villa AM, Ramirez CC. Novel opportunities in the treatment and prevention of scarring. J Cutan Med Surg 2004;8(Suppl 3):32–6.

48. Berman B, Flores F. Recurrence rates of excised keloids treated with postoperative triamcinolone acetonide injections or interferon alfa-2b injections. J Am Acad Dermatol 1997;27:755–7.

49. Berman B, Perez OA, Konda S, et al. A review of the biologic effects, clinical efficacy, and safety of silicone elastomer sheeting for hypertrophic and keloid scar treatment and management. Dermatol Surg 2007;33(11):1291–302.

50. Shridharani SM, Magarakis M, Manson PN, et al. The emerging role of antineoplastic agents in the treatment of keloids and hypertrophic scars: a review. Ann Plast Surg 2010;64(3):355–61.

51. Aggarwal H, Saxena A, Lubana PS, et al. Treatment of keloids and hypertrophic scars using bleomycin. J Cosmet Dermatol 2008;7:43–9.

52. Saray Y, Gulec AT. Treatment of keloids and hypertrophic scars with dermojet injections of bleomycin: a preliminary study. Int J Dermatol 2005;44: 777–84.

53. Stewart CE 4th, Kim JY. Application of mitomycin-C for head and neck keloids. Otolaryngol Head Neck Surg 2006;135(6):946–50.

54. Bailey JN, Waite AE, Clayton WJ, et al. Application of topical mitomycin C to the base of shave-removed keloid scars to prevent their recurrence. Br J Dermatol 2007;156:682–6.

55. Wendling J, Marchand A, Mauviel A, et al. 5-fluorouracil blocks transforming growth factor-beta-induced alpha 2 type I collagen gene (COL1A2) expression in human fibroblasts via c-Jun NH2-terminal kinase/activator protein-1 activation. Mol Pharmacol 2003;64:707–14.

56. Kontochristopoulos G, Stefanaki C, Panagiotopoulos A, et al. Intralesional 5-fluorouracil in the treatment of keloids: an open clinical and histopathologic study. J Am Acad Dermatol 2005;52:474–9.

57. Haurani MJ, Foreman K, Yang JJ, et al. 5-Fluorouracil treatment of problematic scars. Plast Reconstr Surg 2009;123:139–48 [discussion: 149–51].

58. Wang XQ, Liu YK, Wang ZY, et al. Antimitotic drug injections and radiotherapy: a review of the effectiveness of treatment for hypertrophic scars and keloids. Int J Low Extrem Wounds 2008;7(3):151–9.

59. Darougheh A, Asilian A, Shariati F. Intralesional triamcinolone alone or in combination with 5-fluorouracil for the treatment of keloid and hypertrophic scars. Clin Exp Dermatol 2009;34(2):219–23.

Enhancement of Facial Scars With Dermabrasion

Joshua B. Surowitz, MD[a],*, William W. Shockley, MD[b]

KEYWORDS

- Dermabrasion • Wound healing • Facial scars
- Facial trauma

Dermabrasion is a well-established method of skin resurfacing, used for both facial rejuvenation and scar revision. The earliest known use of dermabrasion dates back to Egypt, 1500 BC, when sandpaper was used to revise scars.[1] Many forms of skin resurfacing are available, including chemical peels, laser resurfacing, and mechanical resurfacing, known as *dermabrasion*. Dermabrasion results in the removal of the epidermis along with partial removal of the dermis. Dermabrasion devices consist of a powered hand piece and either a wire brush or diamond fraise. Although not viewed as "high tech" or glamorous, dermabrasion continues to be a popular adjunct to scar revision, with many benefits over other resurfacing options. As with any procedure, technical proficiency, experience, and understanding of its applications and limitations are paramount.

PHYSIOLOGY OF WOUND HEALING

Understanding the physiology of wound healing is important when considering any skin resurfacing procedure. Wound healing occurs in progressive phases: the inflammatory phase, the proliferative phase, and the maturation phase; with significant overlap between the inflammatory and proliferative phases (**Fig. 1**).

Inflammatory Phase

During the inflammatory phase, injury to endothelial cells results in exposure of subendothelial collagen, which acts as a binding surface for aggregation of platelets and results in their activation. The extrinsic and intrinsic coagulation cascades then occur, ultimately resulting in the activation of thrombin, which converts fibrinogen to fibrin. Fibrin then acts as the substrate for further platelet aggregation, migration of inflammatory cells, and plasma proteins. The inflammatory phase initially involves a period of vasoconstriction, mediated by epinephrine, norepinephrine, prostaglandins, serotonin, and thromboxane. This stage is followed by vasodilation, which is activated by histamines, prostaglandins, kinins, and leukotrienes. Macrophages function in phagocytosis and also release chemotactic and growth factors, including transforming growth factor (TGF)-β, basic fibroblast growth factor, epidermal growth factor, TGF-α, and platelet-derived growth factor, which is critical in endothelial cell and fibroblast proliferation.[2–4]

Proliferative Phase

The proliferative phase begins within 24 hours of injury and has significant overlap with the inflammatory phase. Epithelial regeneration, fibroplasia, collagen formation, wound contraction, and neovascularization all occur during the proliferative phase. Epithelial regeneration begins within 24 hours of injury and is at its peak between 48 and 72 hours.[5] Reepithelialization occurs as a result of the migration of epithelial cells from the wound margins and from within adnexal

The authors have no conflicts of interest and nothing to disclose.

[a] Department of Otolaryngology/Head and Neck Surgery, University of North Carolina at Chapel Hill, G190, Physician's Office Building, CB 7070, Chapel Hill, NC 27599, USA

[b] Facial Plastic and Reconstructive Surgery, Department of Otolaryngology/Head and Neck Surgery, University of North Carolina School of Medicine, CB # 7070, G105 Physicians Office Building, 170 Manning Drive, Chapel Hill, NC 27599-7070, USA

* Corresponding author.

E-mail address: JSurowit@unch.unc.edu

Facial Plast Surg Clin N Am 19 (2011) 517–525

doi:10.1016/j.fsc.2011.05.013

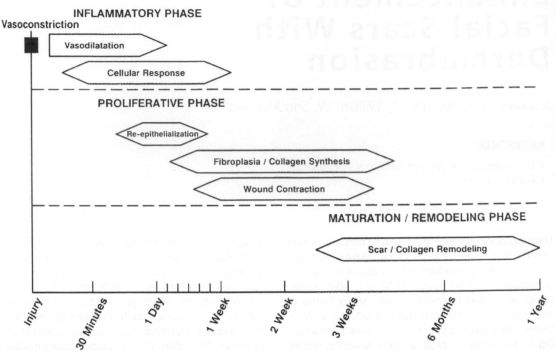

Fig. 1. Phases of wound healing. (*From* Fisher E, Frodel J. Wound healing. In: Papel I, editor. Facial plastic and reconstructive surgery. New York: Thieme; 2009. p. 17; with permission.)

structures of the skin, which include sweat glands, hair follicles, and sebaceous glands.[2,6] Basal stem cells within the adnexae undergo differentiation and subsequent migration, which is why it is paramount to dermabrade only down as far as the superficial reticular dermis, otherwise epithelialization will be impaired and scarring may result (**Fig. 2**).[5] Apposition of advancing epithelial cells results in inhibition of further migration, and in stratification and differentiation.

Fibroplasia, which is the growth of fibroblasts within the wound, occurs 48 to 72 hours after injury and is associated with a significant increase in collagen synthesis, which is most prominent 4 days after injury.[5,7] In addition to collagen, fibroblasts also secrete elastin, fibronectin, glycosaminoglycans, and collagenase. Granulation tissue and neovascularization are also noted during the proliferative phase. Granulation tissue forms during the reepithelialization process, usually beginning at day 3 or 4, and continues until reepithelialization is complete. Wound contraction occurs as fibroblasts differentiate into myofibroblasts, reaching its maximum around 10 to 15 days after injury.[5]

Maturation Phase

The maturation or remodeling phase begins approximately 3 weeks after injury. During this phase, type III collagen is replaced by type I collagen, with reorientation of collagen fibers parallel to the scar, and regression of neovascularization. Scar tensile strength is ultimately 70% to 80% of that encountered in nonwounded skin.[8,9] The maturation phase can take up to 18 months after injury.

Yarborough[10] proposed that dermabrasion created a reorientation of collagen fibers parallel to the lines of wound tension, which may account for some of the scar contour smoothing effects noted after the procedure. Harmon and colleagues[11] performed ultrastructural evaluation of scars resulting from excision and primary closure of cutaneous malignancies in patients who underwent primary closure and those who underwent primary closure with dermabrasion. Serial punch biopsies over the course of 6 weeks showed organized unidirectional collagen fiber orientation parallel to the epidermal surface in the dermabrasion specimens, whereas the control specimens were found to have more-sparse and less-well-organized collagen fiber orientation.

PREOPERATIVE CONSIDERATIONS

Surgeons should obtain a complete past medical history, including a current list of all medications, especially anticoagulants. Patients taking anticoagulants should discontinue these 2 weeks before dermabrasion if medically feasible. Acne scarring is

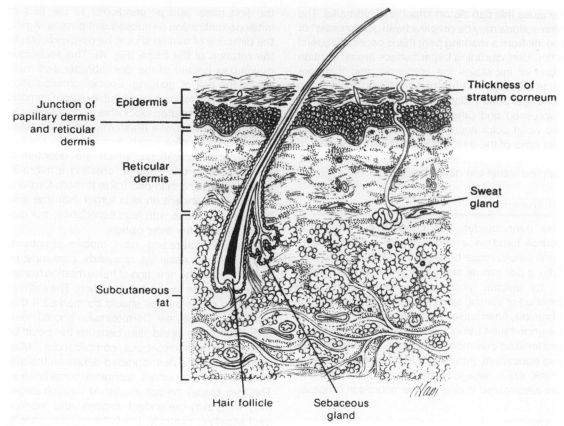

Fig. 2. Normal anatomy of the skin and appendages. (*From* Fisher E, Frodel J. Wound healing. In: Papel I, editor. Facial plastic and reconstructive surgery. New York: Thieme; 2009. p. 16; with permission.)

a common indication for dermabrasion, and therefore it is important to ask about recent or current use of isotretinoin (13-cis-retinoic acid; Accutane). Because of concerns regarding hypertrophic scarring and keloid formation, patients taking isotretinoin should discontinue this 6 to 12 months before dermabrasion.[12] Hydroquinone and retinoic acid may be prescribed to help prevent hyperpigmentation after dermabrasion.[13–17] Hydroquinone inhibits melanocyte conversion of tyrosine to 3,4-dihydroxyphenylalanine and is typically prescribed as a 4% topical cream or gel applied twice daily.[18] Retinoic acid (0.05% cream applied once daily) started 2 weeks before dermabrasion was shown by Mandy[19] to result in expedited reepithelialization. Additionally, he found that no patients who resumed once-daily topical 0.05% retinoic acid within 1 week of dermabrasion experienced postoperative postinflammatory hyperpigmentation or milia compared with 28% in the control group.[19] Prophylaxis against herpes simplex virus (HSV) outbreak should be considered in patients with a history to prevent reactivation. The authors do not typically use any preoperative medications

when performing dermabrasion for a limited facial scar.

DERMABRASION
Anesthesia

For traumatic and surgical scars, local anesthesia is preferred. The local anesthetic is injected into the dermis surrounding the scar and into the scar itself. The authors typically use a lidocaine with epinephrine solution. The injection provides tissue turgor, and the epinephrine minimizes oozing. Regional blocks may also be used, especially if a larger surface area is to be addressed.

Skin Preparation

Proper skin tumescence helps maintain a uniform depth of dermabrasion and maximizes the surgeon's control of the dermabrader. Several methods can be used to accomplish this, including skin refrigerants, infiltration with local anesthetic, and mechanically stretching the skin surface to create skin tension. Special care must be undertaken when infiltrating with local anesthetic, because this can distort important landmarks. The skin surface may be prepared with gentian violet or the ink from a marking pen; this is especially useful when dermabrading larger surface areas. Gentian violet or ink stains the epidermis, and therefore once the epidermis has been removed the surgeon no longer sees violet stain. In treating the multiple depressed and pitted scars resulting from acne, the violet color accentuates these areas after the first pass of the dermabrader. The surgeon should avoid using gauze, because it may become tangled within the dermabrader.

Equipment

The dermabrader unit consists of the power source, hand piece, and cord (**Fig. 3**). Dermabrader hand pieces rotate between 10,000 to 50,000 revolutions per minute and are powered pneumatically or by electric motor. Diamond fraises or wire brushes of varying sizes are used to perform dermabrasion. Alternatively, manual dermabrasion may be undertaken using a wire brush, diamond fraise, or sterilized common sandpaper. Personal protective equipment, including eye protection and facemask, are a necessity, because blood and tissue are aerosolized during the dermabrasion process.

Technique

The dermabrader may be held like a pencil or with all four fingers around the handpiece, with the thumb toward the neck. The latter method was advocated by Yarborough[20] when using the wire brush, because it affords better control and minimizes the risk of ricochet of the device. This method is also used by the authors, although they typically use a diamond fraise. Yarborough[20] recommends pulling the wire brush in a unidirectional fashion and perpendicular to the plane of rotation. Bradley and Park[21] advocate that stroke direction should be 45° to the axis of the scar on

the first pass, and perpendicular to the axis of initial dermabrasion on subsequent passes. Again, the direction of motion should be perpendicular to the rotation of the fraise (**Fig. 4**). This technique maximizes control of the dermabrader and minimizes the risk of gouging. Special consideration must be given to the type of fraise used. Diamond fraises may be rotated clockwise or counterclockwise, whereas the wire brush may only be rotated clockwise.[20,22] Wire brush dermabrasion creates microscopic lacerations, which are oriented at right angles to one another, creating a micro-Z-plasty effect. The diamond fraise is more forgiving and less dependent on skin turgor than the wire brush.[22] For those with less experience, the diamond fraise is the safer option.

When dermabrading near mobile structures, such as the lip, nasal ala, or eyelids, care must be taken to orient the direction of fraise rotation toward these structures to prevent distortion. The esthetic boundary of the eyelids should be marked if they are in the field of view. Dermabrasion should never encroach on the eyelid skin, because this could be associated with disastrous complications. Minimizing blood and dermabraded debris on the skin surface is an important technical consideration. The former may be accomplished through beginning in gravity-dependent regions and working cephalically or centrally. The latter requires consideration of the direction of rotation of the fraise. As advocated by Bradley and Park,[21] moving a fraise rotating in the clockwise direction from left to right will result in deposition of debris behind the path of abrasion.

Diffuse pinpoint bleeding heralds entry into the papillary dermis (**Fig. 5B**). A yellow chamois color marks the reticular dermis, with the superficial reticular dermis characterized by parallel oriented strands, and the deeper reticular dermis by frayed

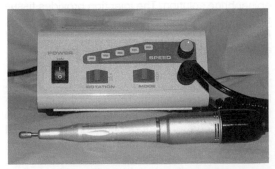

Fig. 3. Dermabrader instrument demonstrating power source, cord, and dermabrader handle. A diamond fraise is attached.

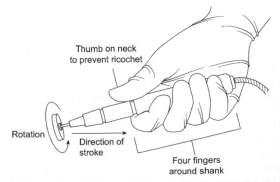

Thumb on neck to prevent ricochet

Rotation

Direction of stroke

Four fingers around shank

Fig. 4. Dermabrader motion should remain perpendicular to the direction of fraise rotation. (*From* Yarborough JM Jr. Dermabrasion by wire brush. J Dermatol Surg Oncol 1987;13(6):610–5; with permission.)

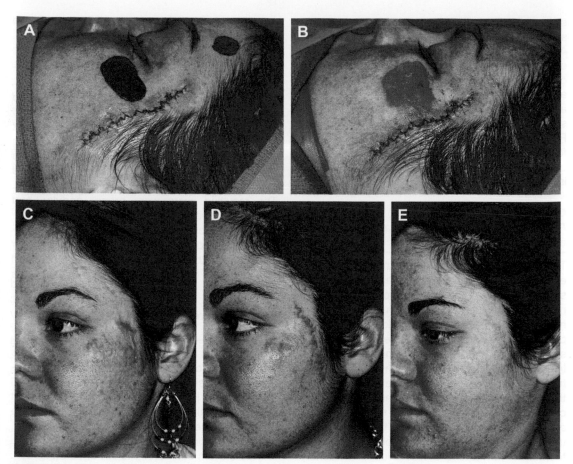

Fig. 5. (*A*) Scars over left cheek and left forehead covered with ink from a marking pen. Adjacent skin shows immediate result after scar revision with geometric broken line closure. (*B*) Punctate bleeding noted in areas of dermabrasion. (*C*) Preoperative photograph showing irregular scars over the left cheek and left forehead and a hypertrophic left preauricular scar. (*D*) Early result (3 weeks) after dermabrasion and preauricular scar revision. (*E*) Results at 6 months after dermabrasion and scar revision.

white strands. Entry into the deep reticular dermis should be avoided because it is associated with scarring.[23] Careful depth control spares stem cells located within the adnexal structures that lie within the reticular dermis.

POSTOPERATIVE CARE

Counseling patients regarding proper postoperative care is critical. Reepithelialization has been shown in animal models to be expedited through maintaining a moist wound, which optimizes epithelial migration,[24] and is maximized by using ointment or occlusive dressings. Complete reepithelialization usually occurs within 7 to 10 days after dermabrasion. Wounds may be left open or managed with occlusive dressings. Wounds left open require meticulous postoperative care involving frequent cleansing with mild soap and water, followed by application of ointment.

Occlusive dressings such as Vigilon (Bard Inc, Murray Hill, NJ, USA) have been shown to result in wounds that heal more rapidly and with less crusting than those left open.[25] After segmental or limited dermabrasion, the authors typically manage wounds in an open fashion with frequent cleansing followed by application of a mild ointment. Sun avoidance and frequent application of sunscreen are paramount. Erythema is expected, commonly lasts for weeks to months, and generally resolves with time.[21] If necessary, topical or systemic steroids can be used to decrease erythema in the postoperative period.[26]

TIMING OF DERMABRASION

The timing of dermabrasion is variable. Yarborough[10] advocated early dermabrasion, ideally between 4 and 8 weeks postinjury. They theorized that scars treated earlier than 4 weeks had a tendency to spread, because they lacked appropriate tensile strength. Katz and Oca[27] studied wound healing at 4, 6, and 8 weeks postinjury using diamond fraise dermabrasion, and reported the most optimal outcomes at 8 weeks. The authors theorized that an 8-week-old scar had more tensile strength than a 4- or 6-week-old scar, and consequently responded better to dermabrasion. Brenner and Perro[18] recommended that dermabrasion be performed 6 to 12 weeks after closure or reconstruction of skin cancer defects, because collagen remodeling is active during this time-frame.

CASE STUDIES
Patient 1: Facial Trauma: Lacerations and Deep Abrasions

This patient is a 22-year-old woman who experienced facial lacerations and deep abrasions resulting from a motor vehicle accident. Areas of modest soft tissue loss also occurred. These areas healed through secondary intention. At 2 months postinjury, she was noted to have broad irregular scars involving the left cheek and left forehead. In addition, she had a 5.5 × 0.8 cm left preauricular hypertrophic scar. At 6 months after her injuries, the patient underwent dermabrasion of the left cheek and forehead scars. At the same time, a scar revision was performed for the left preauricular scar using the geometric broken line closure technique. A marking pen was used to identify the confines of the left cheek and forehead scars before dermabrasion (**Fig. 6**A). Dermabrasion was performed to the level of punctate bleeding

(see **Fig. 6**B). The preoperative and postoperative results are shown in **Fig. 6**C–E.

Patient 2: Facial Trauma: Multiple Facial Lacerations and Foreign Bodies

This patient is a 13-year-old girl who was involved in a motor vehicle accident. Her injuries included multiple facial lacerations involving the right cheek and periorbital region. Multiple glass fragments were imbedded in the soft tissues. Foreign bodies were removed and the wounds were irrigated. The lacerations were closed primarily (see **Fig. 5**A). The resulting scars were broad, nodular, and hyperemic (see **Fig. 5**B). Dermabrasion was performed 24 months after the initial injury and resulted in improvement in the texture and contour of the skin, although persistent erythema was still visible at 6 months after dermabrasion (see **Fig. 5**C).

Patient 3: Facial Trauma: Extensive Soft Tissue Injury

This patient is a 51-year-old man who is a tattoo artist. He lost control of his motorcycle and experienced extensive soft tissue injuries, including full thickness skin loss over the nasal dorsum and right forehead. Multiple reconstructive procedures were required for these defects and the resulting scars. One of his posttraumatic deformities included a wide 5.5-cm scar over the left cheek (**Fig. 7**A). At 3 months after his injury, a scar revision procedure was performed, consisting of excision of the scar and repair with a running W-plasty (see

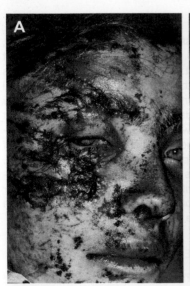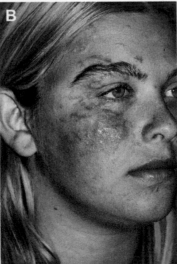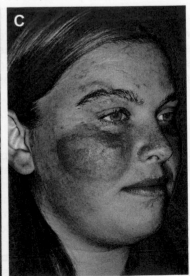

Fig. 6. (A) Multiple facial lacerations immediately after primary repair. (B) Broad irregular scars involving right cheek and right periorbital region 10 months after the initial injury. (C) Improved contour and texture of right cheek 6 months after dermabrasion with mild persistent erythema.

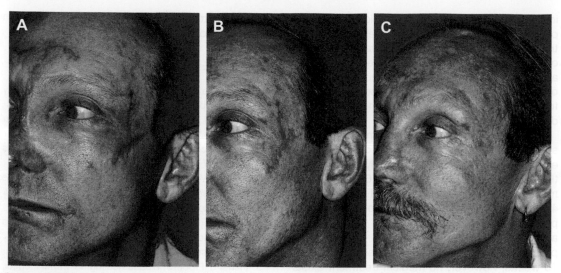

Fig. 7. (*A*) Wide erythematous scar left cheek. (*B*) Early result after excision with W-plasty scar revision. (*C*) Final result 1 year after scar revision and dermabrasion (performed 3 months after scar revision).

Fig. 7B). The resultant scar was further improved with dermabrasion, performed 3 months after the scar revision, at the time of other reconstructive procedures (see **Fig. 7**C).

COMPLICATIONS OF DERMABRASION

The most dreaded and avoidable complication of dermabrasion is scarring. Scarring is caused by working too deeply, which damages adnexal structures and compromises the reepithelialization process.

Hypertrophic scarring and keloid formation are potential complications, and therefore it is important to ask patients about any history of structures such as surgical scars or traumatic scars. **Fig. 8**A illustrates a patient with perioral rhytids who developed hypertrophic scar formation after dermabrasion by a colleague of the senior author. **Fig. 8**B shows improvement of perioral rhytids with

postoperative hypertrophic scar formation, which was ultimately excised and closed primarily.

Concern also exists regarding the effect of isotretinoin on hypertrophic scar and keloid formation because of its suppressive effect on the sebaceous glands.[28–30] Sebaceous glands play a critical role in the reepithelialization process. Studies by Rubenstein and colleagues[31] in 1986 and Katz and colleagues[32] in 1994 showed poor outcomes (ie, hypertrophic scarring and keloid formation) after dermabrasion in the setting of recent isotretinoin use. Rivera[12] advocated stopping isotretinoin at least 6 to 12 months before any planned dermabrasion. More recently, Bagatin and colleagues[33] performed manual dermabrasion (not powered) using a diamond fraise on seven patients, all actively taking oral isotretinoin at dermabrasion. They observed no abnormal scarring or keloid formation in this study population, and suggested that the immunologic and

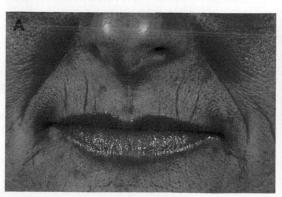
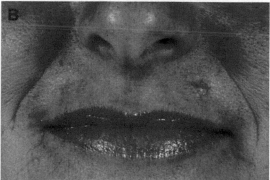

Fig. 8. (*A*) Preoperative photograph showing perioral rhytids before dermabrasion. (*B*) Postoperative result showing improvement of perioral rhytids with development of hypertrophic scar on left upper lip.

inflammatory response may play more of a role in postdermabrasion scarring and keloid formation than isotretinoin. Although the literature is equivocal, isotretinoin use warrants special consideration. Until definitive evidence suggests otherwise, the authors advocate discontinuing isotretinoin at least 6 to 12 months before dermabrasion.

Hyperpigmentation is more common in dark-skinned patients, and can be exacerbated by estrogen use and sun exposure. Hyperpigmentation usually resolves within 3 to 6 months and may also be treated with a topical application of 4% hydroquinone and 0.05% retinoic acid. Hypopigmentation usually occurs within 1 to 2 months and is also more common in dark-skinned patients. This effect will usually resolve over 6 to 10 weeks; however, no medical treatment exists for hypopigmentation. Makeup may be the only remedy in these circumstances.

Milia is a condition of small inclusion cysts within the epidermis, which can be directly excised and also responds to retinoids. In a prospective series, Mandy[19] noted a significantly lower postoperative incidence of milia (and postinflammatory hyperpigmentation) in patients treated with 0.05% topical retinoic acid applied once daily started within 1 week after dermabrasion compared with controls not given postoperative retinoids.

Patients should also be counseled about the risks of bleeding and infection. The most common infectious organisms are Staphylococcus aureus, HSV, and Candida. Staphylococcal infection most often presents with edema, honey crusting, and fevers within 48 to 72 hours postoperatively. HSV reactivation is recognized as pain disproportionate to the examination within 48 to 72 hours postoperatively. Patients with a known history of HSV infection should be treated prophylactically to prevent reactivation. Valacyclovir (500 mg by mouth twice daily) or similar antiviral medications may be started the day before or the day of surgery, with several studies advocating a 10-day postoperative course.[34–36] Candida infections tend to manifest later, usually at 5 to 7 days, with the hallmarks being delayed healing, edema, and exudates. Eczema and dermatitis occur in up to 10% of patients and can be treated with topical, intralesional, or systemic steroids.[21]

SUMMARY

Dermabrasion remains an effective adjunct to scar revision. It is a well-established technique with well-studied outcomes. In contrast to carbon dioxide laser resurfacing, dermabrasion has lower capital investment costs, lower maintenance costs, a better safety profile, and can be used in almost any outpatient setting.

REFERENCES

1. Lawrence N, Mandy S, Yarborough J, et al. History of dermabrasion. Dermatol Surg 2000;26(2):95–101.
2. Goslen J. Physiology of wound healing and scar formation. In: Thomas J, Holt G, editors. Facial scars: incision, revision, and camouflage. St Louis (MO): CV Mosby; 1989. p. 12.
3. Kanzler MH, Gorsulowsky DC, Swanson NA. Basic mechanisms in the healing cutaneous wound. J Dermatol Surg Oncol 1986;12(11):1156–64.
4. Pierce GF. Macrophages: important physiologic and pathologic sources of polypeptide growth factors. Am J Respir Cell Mol Biol 1990;2(3):233–4.
5. Fisher E, Frodel J. Wound healing. In: Papel I, editor. Facial plastic and reconstructive surgery. New York: Thieme; 2009. p. 15–25.
6. Krawczyk WS. A pattern of epidermal cell migration during wound healing. J Cell Biol 1971;49(2): 247–63.
7. Gourin C, Terris D. Dynamics of wound healing. In: Bailey B, Johnson J, editors. Head and neck surgery—otolaryngology. Philadelphia: Lippincott Williams & Wilkins; 2006. p. 197–213.
8. Goslen JB. Wound healing for the dermatologic surgeon. J Dermatol Surg Oncol 1988;14(9):959–72.
9. Levenson SM, Geever EF, Crowley LV, et al. The healing of rat skin wounds. Ann Surg 1965;161:293–308.
10. Yarborough JM Jr. Ablation of facial scars by programmed dermabrasion. J Dermatol Surg Oncol 1988;14(3):292–4.
11. Harmon CB, Zelickson BD, Roenigk RK, et al. Dermabrasive scar revision. Immunohistochemical and ultrastructural evaluation. Dermatol Surg 1995; 21(6):503–8.
12. Rivera AE. Acne scarring: a review and current treatment modalities. J Am Acad Dermatol 2008;59(4): 659–76.
13. Spencer M. Topical use of hydroquinone for depigmentation. JAMA 1965;194(9):962–4.
14. Palumbo A, d'Ischia M, Misuraca G, et al. Mechanism of inhibition of melanogenesis by hydroquinone. Biochim Biophys Acta 1991;1073(1):85–90.
15. Grimes PE. Management of hyperpigmentation in darker racial ethnic groups. Semin Cutan Med Surg 2009;28(2):77–85.
16. Ortonne JP. Retinoic acid and pigment cells: a review of in-vitro and in-vivo studies. Br J Dermatol 1992; 127(Suppl 41):43–7.
17. Kaplan B, Potter T, Moy RL. Scar revision. Dermatol Surg 1997;23(6):435–42 [quiz: 443–4].
18. Brenner MJ, Perro CA. Recontouring, resurfacing, and scar revision in skin cancer reconstruction. Facial Plast Surg Clin North Am 2009;17(3):469–87, e3.

19. Mandy SH. Tretinoin in the preoperative and postoperative management of dermabrasion. J Am Acad Dermatol 1986;15(4 Pt 2):878–9, 888–9.

20. Yarborough JM Jr. Dermabrasion by wire brush. J Dermatol Surg Oncol 1987;13(6):610–5.

21. Bradley DT, Park SS. Scar revision via resurfacing. Facial Plast Surg 2001;17(4):253–62.

22. Alt TH. Facial dermabrasion: advantages of the diamond fraise technique. J Dermatol Surg Oncol 1987; 13(6):618–24.

23. Koranda F. Dermabrasion. In: Thomas JR, Roller J, editors. Cutaneous facial surgery. New York: Thieme; 1992. p. 104.

24. Winter GD. Formation of the scab and the rate of epithelization of superficial wounds in the skin of the young domestic pig. Nature 1962;193:293–4.

25. Mandy SH. A new primary wound dressing made of polyethylene oxide gel. J Dermatol Surg Oncol 1983;9(2):153–5.

26. Bernstein LJ, Kauvar AN, Grossman MC, et al. The short- and long-term side effects of carbon dioxide laser resurfacing. Dermatol Surg 1997;23(7): 519–25.

27. Katz BE, Oca AG. A controlled study of the effectiveness of spot dermabrasion ('scarabrasion') on the appearance of surgical scars. J Am Acad Dermatol 1991;24(3):462–6.

28. Goldstein JA, Comite H, Mescon H, et al. Isotretinoin in the treatment of acne: histologic changes, sebum production, and clinical observations. Arch Dermatol 1982;118(8):555–8.

29. Nelson AM, Zhao W, Gilliland KL, et al. Early gene changes induced by isotretinoin in the skin provide clues to its mechanism of action. Dermatoendocrinol 2009;1(2):100–1.

30. Nelson AM, Zhao W, Gilliland KL, et al. Temporal changes in gene expression in the skin of patients treated with isotretinoin provide insight into its mechanism of action. Dermatoendocrinol 2009;1(3): 177–87.

31. Rubenstein R, Roenigk HH Jr, Stegman SJ, et al. Atypical keloids after dermabrasion of patients taking isotretinoin. J Am Acad Dermatol 1986; 15(2 Pt 1):280–5.

32. Katz BE, Mac Farlane DF. Atypical facial scarring after isotretinoin therapy in a patient with previous dermabrasion. J Am Acad Dermatol 1994;30(5 Pt 2):852–3.

33. Bagatin E, dos Santos Guadanhim LR, Yarak S, et al. Dermabrasion for acne scars during treatment with oral isotretinoin. Dermatol Surg 2010;36(4):483–9.

34. Gilbert S, McBurney E. Use of valacyclovir for herpes simplex virus-1 (HSV-1) prophylaxis after facial resurfacing: a randomized clinical trial of dosing regimens. Dermatol Surg 2000;26(1):50–4.

35. Beeson WH, Rachel JD. Valacyclovir prophylaxis for herpes simplex virus infection or infection recurrence following laser skin resurfacing. Dermatol Surg 2002;28(4):331–6.

36. Gilbert S. Improving the outcome of facial resurfacing—prevention of herpes simplex virus type 1 reactivation. J Antimicrob Chemother 2001;47(Suppl T1): 29–34.

Laser Treatment for Improvement and Minimization of Facial Scars

Joseph F. Sobanko, MD[a],*, Tina S. Alster, MD[b]

KEYWORDS

- Scar revision • Laser treatment • Fractionated laser
- Pulsed dye laser

Take-home points: Scar formation and revision

- An imbalance in wound-healing homeostasis is at the epicenter of scar formation
- Scars, particularly facial scars, significantly affect the lives of patients
- Physicians can improve the quality of patients' lives via scar revision
- Numerous scar treatments are available, but lasers have proven to deliver the most reproducibly good results

---

The psychosocial impact of cutaneous scarring can be profound. Scars inflicted by traumatic incidents, surgical procedures, and severe acne bear a heavy emotional burden on patients, particularly when present on visible areas such as the face.[1–3] The quality of life of patients may be affected from aesthetic concerns in addition to chronic symptoms such as pruritus and pain.[4] In addition, substantial anxiety and self-consciousness has been noted in men and women when trauma or elective procedures result in even nominal scarring.[3,5] Cutaneous injuries that result in scar tissue formation are relatively common and lead patients to seek treatment for cosmetic or functional improvement. It is imperative for physicians to recognize that physical improvement of scars can translate into improved psychosocial well-being and behavior of patients.[6,7]

Scars are the result of a deviation in the orderly pattern of healing and can be caused by a variety of factors, such as excessive wound tension, improper surgical repair, delayed reepithelialization, or a history of radiation to the affected area. The underlying pathophysiologic mechanism appears to be an imbalance of matrix degradation and collagen biosynthesis.[8] An overzealous healing response can create a raised nodule of fibrotic tissue, whereas "pitted" and atrophic scars may result from inadequate replacement of deleted collagen fibers. Although vascular and pigment alterations associated with wound healing are typically transient, the textural changes caused by collagen disruption are often permanent. Histologically, what makes scars unique is the relative absence of skin appendages and elastic fibers—constituents of normal skin that may account for the loss of flexibility seen in scar tissue.[9]

There are several currently available scar-reducing therapies and many other agents that

---

Author disclosures: None relevant to this article.
a Perelman Center for Advanced Medicine, University of Pennsylvania, 3400 Civic Center Boulevard, Room 1-330S, Philadelphia, PA 19104, USA
b Washington Institute of Dermatologic Laser Surgery, 1430 K Street, North West Suite 200, Washington, DC 20005, USA
* Corresponding author.
E-mail address: joseph.sobanko@gmail.com

Facial Plast Surg Clin N Am 19 (2011) 527–542
doi:10.1016/j.fsc.2011.06.006

may emerge to have the potential to eliminate scarring.[10-12] Some of the most commonly used modalities to improve scar appearance include intralesional corticosteroids, 5-fluorouracil, and bleomycin. It is likely that these agents exert their effect on scars by suppressing inflammation and/or collagen production.[13-15] Combination therapy is often advocated as a means of increasing efficacy and decreasing total medication dosage, thereby decreasing the likelihood of adverse effects.[16,17] Radiation therapy and surgical intervention, particularly in combination with one another, are sometimes used for refractory and recurrent scars.[18] Unfortunately, each of these methods has been associated with unacceptably high incidences of scar recurrence and other untoward sequelae such as skin atrophy, dyspigmentation, and pain. Laser scar revision is a safe procedure with clinically demonstrable efficacy and minimal side effects that may be used in combination with the aforementioned scar treatments. The remainder of this article addresses the use of lasers for the treatment of scars.

HISTORY OF LASER SCAR REVISION

> **Take-home points: Overview of laser scar revision**
>
> - The principles of selective photothermolysis help guide the laser surgeon in choosing the proper laser wavelength and treatment parameters for scar revision
> - Proper scar classification is essential for optimizing treatment results

Although laser surgery is more than 5 decades old, the field was revolutionized in 1983 when Anderson and Parrish[19] elucidated the principles of selective photothermolysis. This basic theory of laser-tissue interaction explains how selective tissue destruction is possible. To effect precise thermal destruction of target tissue without unwanted conduction of heat to surrounding structures, the proper laser wavelength must be selected for preferential absorption by the intended tissue chromophore. Furthermore, the pulse duration of laser emission must be shorter than the thermal relaxation time of the target, thermal relaxation time (T_R) being defined as the amount of time necessary for the targeted structure to cool to one-half of its peak temperature immediately after laser irradiation. The delivered fluence (energy density) must also be sufficiently high to cause the desired degree of thermal injury to the skin. Thus the laser wavelength, pulse duration, and fluence must each be carefully chosen to achieve maximal target ablation while minimizing surrounding tissue damage.

Laser systems are versatile tools that allow for a broad range of cutaneous maladies to be treated. Scar improvement with a pulsed dye laser (PDL) was first reported in 1993,[20] and over the past decade laser scar revision has progressed tremendously, due to advances in technology.

Laser treatment of scars is optimized by proper scar categorization. Several qualities of the scar including size, color, texture, and prior treatments influence choice of laser wavelength and treatment parameters.

SCAR CLASSIFICATION

> **Take-home points: Clinical appearance of scars**
>
> - Categorization of scars by clinical appearance can be difficult, but is a helpful guide to proper laser treatment
> - Although similar in many respects, hypertrophic scars and keloids should be distinguished from one another to optimize clinical outcome
> - Atrophic scars are dermal depressions and result in significant contour abnormalities
> - Recognition of skin prone to scarring is one tool of evaluation that can be helpful in scar prevention

Numerous scar classification system and evaluation tools have been described.[21-24] At present, no universal model for objective scar assessment has been accepted.[25] In medical literature, scars are often analyzed by their etiology, the most common sources being surgery, trauma, burns, and acne or inflammatory processes. For the purposes of practicality and ease in treatment selection, the authors advocate scar classification as determined by clinical appearance rather than by causation.

Hypertrophic scars are erythematous, raised, firm nodular growths that occur more commonly in areas subject to increased pressure or movement or in body sites that exhibit slow wound healing. The growth of hypertrophic scars is limited to the site of original tissue injury, unlike *keloids*, which proliferate beyond the boundaries of the initial wound and often continue to grow without regression. Keloids present as deep reddish-purple papules and nodules, often on the earlobes, anterior chest, shoulders, and upper back. These lesions are more common in darker-skinned persons and, like hypertrophic scars, may be pruritic, dysesthetic, and cosmetically disfiguring. Whereas the histology of hypertrophic scars is indistinguishable from that of other scarring processes, keloidal histology may be recognized by thickened bundles of hyalinized acellular collagen haphazardly arranged in whorls and nodules with an increased amount of hyaluronidase.[11]

Atrophic scars, on the other hand, are dermal depressions that result from an acute inflammatory process affecting the skin, such as cystic acne or varicella. The inflammation associated with atrophic scars leads to collagen destruction with dermal atrophy. Surgery or other forms of skin trauma may also result in atrophic scars, which are initially erythematous and become increasingly hypopigmented and fibrotic over time. Based on their width, depth, and 3-dimensional architecture, acne scars are sometimes further subclassified into icepick, rolling, and boxcar scars.[26]

Prescars are early wounds in scar-prone skin. Prophylactic or early laser treatment of traumatized skin concomitant with or shortly after cutaneous wounding has been shown to reduce or even prevent scar formation in patients at high risk for scarring.[27–29] Laser therapy may improve the appearance of wounded skin by promoting better collagen organization in healing wounds.[30]

LASER SCAR REVISION
Hypertrophic Scars and Keloids

Take-home points: Pulsed dye laser
• PDL is the laser of choice for hypertrophic scars and keloids, though the mechanism by which it works is yet to be fully elucidated
• PDL may be used alone or in combination with other scar treatments
• PDL is relatively safe, but a series of treatments is often necessary
• The most common adverse events of PDL irradiation are transient purpura and hyperpigmentation

---

Detailed reviews of laser scar revision have previously been published.[31,32] Early in vitro experimentation with a 1064-nm neodymium:yttrium-aluminum-garnet (Nd:YAG) laser demonstrated that fibroblasts irradiated with this wavelength produced decreased amounts of collagen.[33,34] The Nd:YAG, argon, and carbon dioxide (CO_2) lasers were subsequently studied on hypertrophic scars and keloids with early promising results, but high recurrence rates were observed.[35,36] It was not until PDLs were studied that it was shown that scar size, erythema, pliability, pruritus, and texture could be improved.[37–40] A wealth of published clinical data over 2 decades has shown that PDL is effective for all forms of hypertrophic scarring and keloids, regardless of etiology. Burn scars,[39] sternotomy scars,[37] acne scars,[40] and facial scars resulting from cutaneous surgery[29,38] all appear to respond well to PDL. As a consequence of this research, the laser of choice in treating hypertrophic scars and keloids is the vascular-specific 585-nm PDL (**Fig. 1**).[10,32,41]

There is no consensus on the precise mechanism whereby the PDL exerts its effect on scars. The PDL has been demonstrated to reduce expression of transforming growth factor β, fibroblast proliferation, and collagen type III deposition.[42] Other plausible explanations include selective photothermolysis of vasculature,[43] released mast cell constituents (such as histamine and interleukins) that could affect collagen metabolism,[37] and the heating of collagen fibers and breaking of disulfide bonds with subsequent collagen realignment.[39]

Scar revision with the PDL is typically performed on an outpatient basis without anesthesia. All persons present in the room must wear protective eyewear capable of filtering light of 585 to 595 nm to avoid retinal damage.

Any concern regarding patient response to treatment should prompt a test spot or patch in a small area before irradiation of the entire lesion. If postoperative crusting or vesiculation is observed, the fluence applied on subsequent visits should be decreased and retreatment postponed until the skin has completely healed. The fluence and pulse duration can be adjusted if scar proliferation continues despite laser irradiation. Generally speaking, higher fluences and shorter pulse durations result in improved scar size and pliability.[41,44] However, more aggressive laser settings must be carefully considered in patients with darker skin and for scars in more delicate or thin-skinned locations (eg, eyelids, neck, chest).[41,45,46]

The use of concomitant intralesional corticosteroids or 5-fluorouracil has been shown to provide additional benefit in proliferative scars.[47,48] Intralesional injections of corticosteroids (20 mg/mL triamcinolone) are more easily delivered immediately after (rather than before) PDL irradiation because the laser-irradiated scar becomes edematous (making needle penetration easier). An additional consideration is that when steroid injection is performed before laser irradiation the skin blanches, rendering the skin a potentially less amenable target for vascular-specific irradiation.

How I Do It: PDL for hypertrophic scars and keloids

- If topical anesthesia is desired, a lidocaine-containing cream or gel can be applied to the treatment areas 30 to 60 minutes before laser irradiation.
- To avoid interference with laser penetration, the skin should be cleansed with soap and water to remove residual makeup, powder, or creams. Flammable solutions, such as alcohol, should be avoided in skin preparation.
- Wet gauze may be used to protect hair-bearing areas during treatment and to avoid unnecessary thermal injury to nontargeted skin.
- The patient and other individuals present in the treatment room must wear protective eyewear capable of filtering light of 585 to 595 nm to avoid retinal damage.
- The fluences chosen are determined by the skin phototype of the patient, the type of scar, and previous treatments applied to the area.
- It is prudent to begin treatments with the lowest effective energy densities, using increased fluences on subsequent visits only when the response to the previous treatment is suboptimal.
- In general, hypertrophic scars and keloids are treated with moderately low energy densities ranging from 6.0 to 7.5 J/cm^2 when using a spot size of 5 or 7 mm and 4.5 to 5.5 J/cm^2 when using a 10-mm spot size.
- Energy densities should be lowered by at least 0.5 J/cm^2 in patients with darker skin and for scars in more delicate or thin-skinned locations (eg, eyelids, neck, chest).
- Pulse durations ranging from 0.45 to 1.5 milliseconds are commonly used.
- Treat the entire surface of the scar with adjacent, nonoverlapping laser pulses.
- The appearance of most hypertrophic scars will improve by approximately 50% after 2 treatments with the PDL using the aforementioned laser parameters.
- Keloids often require additional treatment sessions to achieve significant improvement, but some may prove altogether unresponsive.
- Laser treatments are typically repeated at 6- to 8-week time intervals.

The most common side effect of treatment with the PDL is postoperative purpura, which often persists for several days. Pulse durations shorter than 6 milliseconds are almost certain to bruise the skin. Edema of treated skin may also occur, but usually subsides within 48 hours. A topical healing ointment under a nonstick bandage can be applied for the first few postoperative days to protect the skin. Treated areas should be gently cleansed daily with water and mild soap. Strict sun avoidance and photoprotection should be advocated between treatment sessions to reduce the risk of pigment alteration. Hyperpigmentation has been reported with varying frequencies (1%–24%).[49,50] If skin darkening occurs, further laser treatment should be suspended until resolution of the dyspigmentation has occurred in order to reduce the risk of cutaneous melanin interference with laser energy penetration. Topical bleaching agents (such as hydroquinone or kojic acid) may be applied to hasten pigment resolution.

Although no studies regarding the use of 532-nm potassium titanyl phosphate (KTP) lasers have been published, some practitioners advocate their use for erythematous scars because of their ability to reduce erythema. Similarly, intense pulsed light systems have been demonstrated to improve scar erythema.[51] The 532-nm frequency-doubled Q-switched Nd:YAG may be used to treat pigmented hypertrophic scars.[52] Vaporization of keloid scars by CO_2 laser irradiation almost universally results in scar recurrences,[53] but there is growing evidence that fractional lasers may improve hypertrophic scarring[54] (see later discussions).

Atrophic Scars

Ablative lasers

Successful recontouring of atrophic scars has been achieved with CO_2 or erbium:yttrium-aluminum-garnet (Er:YAG or erbium) laser vaporization.[55–59] Although other treatments such as dermabrasion and injection of various filler materials can also be used for atrophic scars, their operator-dependent efficacy and side-effect profile, as well as temporary clinical effect (in the case of most filler injections), limit their usefulness and widespread acceptance for the longer term.

Take-home points: Fractional lasers

- Fully ablative and fractional laser systems are the systems of choice to improve atrophic scars
- The choice of laser is primarily determined by the severity of scarring and the patient's ability to tolerate postoperative recovery
- It appears that ablative and nonablative fractional lasers produce similar clinical results to ablative lasers with significantly fewer adverse effects
- The deeper penetration of ablative fractional lasers may lead to enhanced clinical improvement of scars relative to fully ablative and nonablative fractional systems

What popularized laser skin resurfacing treatment for atrophic scar revision was its ability to selectively and reproducibly vaporize skin with improved operator control and clinical efficacy.[60–63] Clinical and histologic comparisons with dermabrasion and chemical peels showed that a predictable amount of skin vaporization and residual thermal damage could only be achieved through lasers, thereby demonstrating the superiority of laser treatment for skin resurfacing.[64]

CO_2 and Er:YAG lasers work to selectively heat and vaporize superficial skin by emitting energy that is absorbed by intracellular tissue water. Cutaneous laser resurfacing produces an additional skin-tightening benefit through controlled heating of dermal collagen. The depth of ablation correlates directly with the number of passes performed, and usually is confined to the epidermis and upper papillary dermis; however, stacking of laser pulses by treating an area with multiple passes in rapid succession or by using a high overlap setting on a scanning device can lead to excessive thermal injury with subsequent increased risk of scarring.[65] An ablative plateau is reached with less effective tissue ablation and accumulation of thermal injury due to reduced tissue water content after initial desiccation. The avoidance of pulse stacking and incomplete removal of partially desiccated tissue is paramount to prevention of excessive thermal accumulation with any laser system. Persistent collagen shrinkage and dermal remodeling are responsible for much of the continued clinical

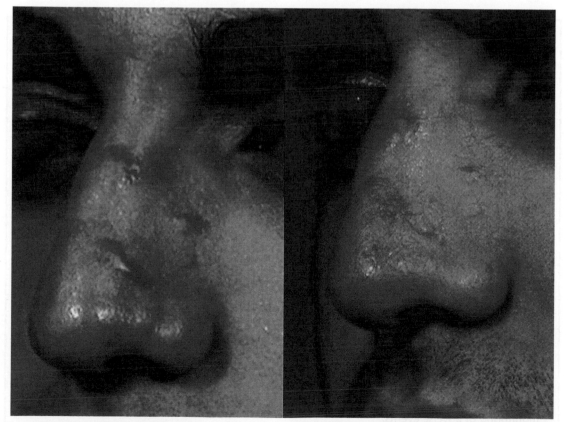

Fig. 1. Hypertrophic scars on the nose before (*left*) and after 2 pulsed dye laser (PDL) treatments (*right*).

benefits observed after ablative laser resurfacing. The photothermal effect of ablative lasers on the skin account for shrinkage of collagen and noticeable clinical skin tightening, as well as neocollagenesis and collagen remodeling that leads to marked reduction of skin textural irregularities.[66]

Laser treatment of atrophic scars is aimed at reducing the depth of the scar borders and stimulating neocollagenesis to fill in the depressions. Although spot (or local) vaporization of isolated scars is a viable treatment option, extended treatment (at least an entire cosmetic unit) is recommended for more widely distributed defects to avoid obvious lines of demarcation between treated and untreated sites. In addition, treatment of a larger surface area increases the overall collagen-tightening effect, thereby improving clinical response by making scars appear shallower.

Absolute contraindications to ablative laser skin resurfacing include an active cutaneous bacterial, viral, or fungal infection. Patients with an inflammatory skin condition (eg, psoriasis, eczema) involving the skin areas to be treated should be avoided. Isotretinoin use within the preceding 6-month period and a history of keloids are also considered contraindications to ablative laser treatment because of the unpredictable tissue-healing response and greater risk for scarring.[67] Ablative laser scar revision is typically performed on an outpatient basis and requires a thoughtful approach by both doctor and patient, including thorough preoperative counseling related to the postoperative recovery period. All persons in the room must be wearing protective eyewear. If patients are wearing protective contact lens shields, sandblasted metal ones must be chosen because plastic shields do not meet safety standards for ocular protection during periocular laser irradiation. The concave surface of the shields should be liberally lubricated with an ophthalmic ointment, and care must be taken while inserting and removing the shields so as to prevent corneal abrasions.

Immediately after ablation the vaporized skin appears erythematous and edematous, with copious serous discharge and generalized worsening of the skin's appearance over the first few days. It is imperative that patients be monitored closely for appropriate healing responses and potential complications, such as dermatitis or infection, during the 7- to 10-day reepithelialization process.[68–70] Full-face procedures or large treatment areas often necessitate the use of prophylactic

---

How I Do It: Ablative lasers for atrophic scars

- The ideal patient for ablative laser skin resurfacing has a fair complexion (skin phototype I or II), although darker skin tones may also be treated.

- Various anesthetic options can be employed, including topical, intralesional, intravenous, and general anesthesia.

- In general, larger treatment areas (eg, full face) require the use of intravenous or general anesthesia for maximal patient comfort.

- Prophylactic antibiotics may be used for full-face procedures or large treatment areas.

- When choosing treatment parameters, the surgeon must consider factors such as the anatomic location to be resurfaced, the skin phototype of the patient, and previous treatments delivered to the area.

- The requisite protective eyewear and other safety precautions (eg, smoke evacuator to capture laser plume) should be used.

- The CO_2 laser is generally used at fluences of 250 to 350 mJ to ablate the epidermis in a single pass.

- Short-pulsed Er:YAG lasers that are operated at 5 to 15 J/cm^2 often require several passes to result in a similar depth of penetration as CO_2, whereas longer-pulsed Er:YAG systems can be operated at higher fluences (22.5 J/cm^2) to achieve comparable results in a single pass.

- Areas with thinner skin (eg, periorbital) require fewer laser passes and nonfacial (eg, neck, chest) laser resurfacing should be avoided, due to the relative paucity of pilosebaceous units in these areas.

- Because of their depth and fibrotic nature, most atrophic scars will require at least 2 laser passes regardless of the laser system chosen for treatment.

- It is important that any partially desiccated tissue be removed with saline-soaked or water-soaked gauze between laser passes for char formation to be avoided.

- Patients should be seen in-office within 24 to 48 hours then at weekly intervals for 1 month for close monitoring of adverse events.

antibiotics and/or antiviral medications to reduce the risk of infection.[71–73] The use of topical antibiotics is avoided because of the potential development of contact dermatitis.[74] Application of topical ointments, semiocclusive dressings, and/or cooling masks promote healing and reduce swelling.

Postoperative erythema typically lasts several weeks after ablative laser treatment, due to tissue necrosis. Hyperpigmentation is transient and generally appears 3 to 4 weeks after treatment. Its resolution can be hastened with the use of topical bleaching agents.[69,70] Although hyperpigmentation is relatively common (particularly in patients with darker skin tones), hypopigmentation is rare.[68] The most severe complications of ablative skin resurfacing include hypertrophic scarring and ectropion formation, both related to overly aggressive laser techniques and/or undiagnosed/ untreated suprainfections.[69,70] Hypertrophic burn scars can be effectively treated with the PDL as previously described,[39] whereas ectropion typically requires surgical reconstruction. Retreatment after ablative laser skin resurfacing should be postponed for at least 1 year to accurately gauge clinical improvement and permit full tissue recovery.[58]

Nonablative lasers

As a consequence of the side effects and prolonged postoperative recovery associated with ablative laser treatment, nonablative lasers were subsequently developed to provide a noninvasive option for atrophic scar revision.[56] The most popular and widely used of these nonablative systems include the 1320-nm Nd:YAG, 1450-nm diode, and 1064-nm Nd:YAG lasers.[75–77] These devices deliver concomitant epidermal surface cooling with deeply penetrating infrared wavelengths that target tissue water and stimulate collagen production via controlled dermal heating without epidermal disruption.[78] A series of 3 to 5 treatments are typically performed on a monthly basis, with optimal clinical efficacy appreciated several (3–6) months after the final laser treatment session. Sustained clinical improvement of scars by 40% to 50% has been observed after the series of treatments.[75–78] The low side-effect profile of these nonablative systems (limited to local erythema and edema and, rarely, vesiculation or herpes simplex reactivation) compensates for their reduced clinical efficacy (relative to ablative lasers).

Fractional lasers

Due to a need for more noticeable clinical improvement than the aforementioned nonablative systems, fractional photothermolysis was developed. In its relatively short history, fractional laser technology has progressed rapidly, with nearly 30 commercially available fractional systems on the market. These laser systems may best be classified into two categories: (1) nonablative fractional lasers (NAFL) and (2) ablative fractional lasers (AFL).[79]

The initial fractional laser (Fraxel; Reliant Technologies, Mountain View, CA, USA) involved the use of a mid-infrared (1550 nm) wavelength erbium-doped fiber laser to create microscopic noncontiguous columns of thermal injury in the dermis (referred to as microscopic thermal zones or MTZs) surrounded by zones of viable tissue. The spatially precise columns of thermal injury produce localized epidermal necrosis and collagen denaturation at 125 or 250 MTZ/cm^2.[80,81] Because the tissue surrounding each MTZ is intact, residual epidermal and dermal cells contribute to rapid healing. Maintenance of the stratum corneum ensures continued epidermal barrier function.

Histologic evaluation of the MTZ demonstrates homogenization of the dermal matrix and the presence of epidermal necrotic debris, representing the extrusion of damaged epidermal keratinocytes by viable keratinocytes at the lateral margin of the MTZ.[81] The necrotic debris exfoliates over the next several days, producing a bronzed appearance to the skin. The wound-healing response differs from that after ablative laser techniques because the epidermal tissue that is spared between thermal zones contains viable transient amplifying cells capable of rapid re-reepithelialization. Furthermore, because the stratum corneum has low water content, it remains intact immediately after treatment. Therefore, the coagulative wound created by NAFL resurfacing is unique and not simply that of an ablative laser used to make "holes" in the skin. In addition, NAFL resurfacing can provide an advantage over purely nonablative laser treatments, due to the gradual exfoliation of the epidermis with resultant improvement in superficial dyspigmentation.[82] A series of NAFL treatments is required to achieve optimal clinical improvement because only a fraction of the skin is treated during a single session.

Significant clinical improvement can be obtained when nonablative fractional photothermolysis is applied to atrophic facial acne scars of mild to moderate severity.[54,83–88] After a series of 3 consecutive NAFL treatments, clinical improvement of 50% or more is observed in acne scarring[83–88] (Fig. 2). Similar results have been obtained in scars resulting from other injuries, including surgery and burns[89–93] (Fig. 3). Patients are treated on a monthly basis, with greater clinical improvement seen with successive treatments. It has been shown that higher energy settings and multiple laser passes translate into improved clinical results while

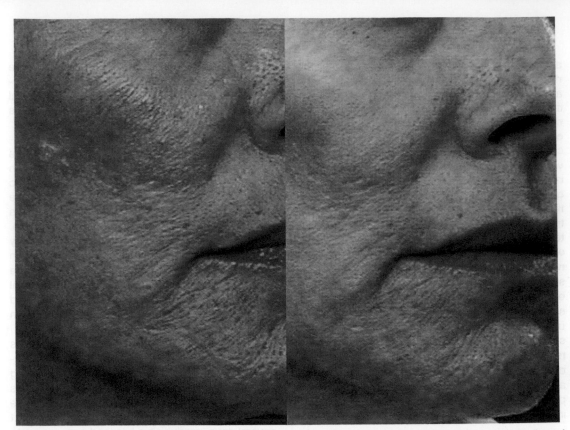

Fig. 2. Atrophic facial acne scars before (*left*) and after 3 consecutive monthly nonablative fractional laser (NAFL) treatments (*right*).

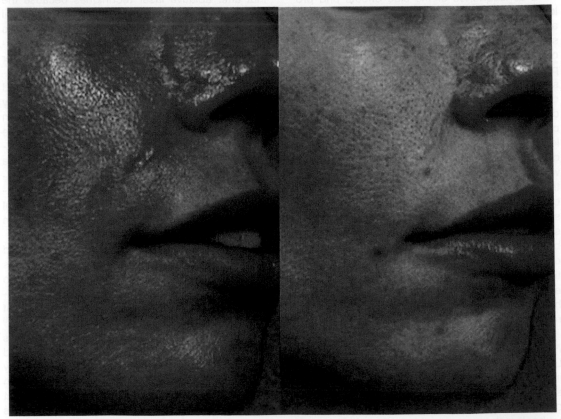

Fig. 3. Surgical facial scar before (*left*) and after one combination 585-nm PDL and NAFL treatment (*right*).

increased density is more likely to result in increased rates and severity of erythema, edema, and hyperpigmentation.[94,95] By contrast, AFLs (fractionated CO_2 and erbium lasers) not only create similar columns of thermal coagulation through the epidermis and dermis, but also vaporize the stratum corneum.[96] Because of the absence of a protective cap overlying the coagulated columnar regions, the immediate postoperative appearance of treated areas appear more similar to an ablative treatment than that observed with NAFL. Unlike fully ablative treatments, AFLs not only deliver sufficient energy to effect immediate contraction, but intact islands of viable epidermis that facilitate rapid healing remain post treatment.[97,98] Intense erythema and serosanguinous drainage are evident for 2 to 3 days, followed by complete re-reepithelialization and diminution of erythema by days 6 or 7.[99]

A variety of atrophic scars on facial and nonfacial skin can be improved significantly by AFL resurfacing techniques[100–107] (**Fig. 4**). Clinical improvement of atrophic scarring results from collagen contraction and neocollagenesis. Given that AFL energy penetrates more deeply (1.5–1.6 mm) into the dermis, it is likely that these systems will prove to be more effective than NAFLs for atrophic scars.[100–107] Thermal burn injuries have also shown textural improvement of skin after AFL treatment.[108]

While the ideal patient for fractional laser skin resurfacing has a fair complexion (skin phototype I, II, or III), darker skin tones (IV–VI) can also be treated. Adequate preoperative patient evaluation and education are necessary to discern unrealistic patient expectations, avoid pitfalls, and optimize clinical outcomes. Prolonged postoperative recovery, pigmentary alteration, or unexpected scarring is much less likely to occur with fractionated technology than with fully ablative lasers, but patients must nevertheless be forewarned. For patients unable or unwilling to withstand the anticipated 3 to 7 days of postoperative healing, a series of nonablative (fractionated or infrared) laser procedures may be a more suitable choice.

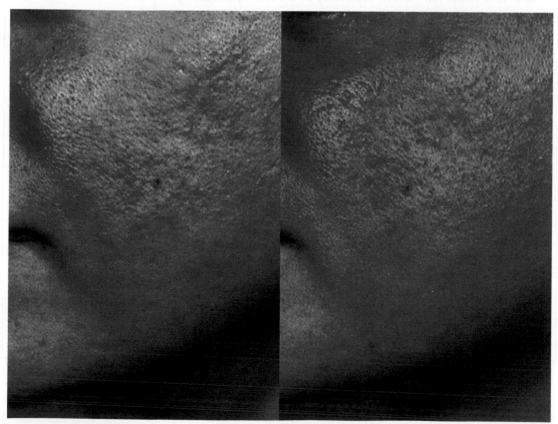

Fig. 4. Atrophic facial acne scars before (*left*) and several months after one ablative fractional laser (AFL) skin resurfacing treatment (*right*).

How I Do It: Fractional lasers for atrophic scars

- The ideal patient for fractional laser skin resurfacing has a fair complexion (skin phototype I, II, or III), but darker skin tones (IV–VI) can also be treated.

- Adequate preoperative patient evaluation and education are essential.

- Sun exposure should be avoided prior to treatment in order to decrease the risk of postoperative dyspigmentation.

- For patients with a strong history of herpes labialis, prophylactic oral antiviral medications should be considered when treating the perioral skin. Reactivation of prior herpes simplex infection can occur despite absence of an external wound, due to the intense dermal heat produced by the laser.

- The treatment areas should be cleansed of debris (including dirt, makeup, and powder) using a mild cleanser and 70% alcohol.

- A topical anesthetic cream is applied to the treatment sites for 60 minutes before treatment. For full-face AFL treatments oral sedation, nerve blocks, tumescent anesthesia, topical anesthetic creams, and intravenous sedation may be required.

- NAFL treatment is delivered concomitantly with forced air cooling. The most commonly used NAFL (Fraxel re:store) is employed at energy settings of 40 to 60 mJ but may be increased to as high as 70 mJ. Total energies of 3 to 5 kJ are typically applied for full-face treatment. Retreatments with gradually higher fluences should be performed at 4-week intervals until patients are satisfied with clinical outcomes (typically 3 to 5 sessions are necessary to produce substantial clinical improvement).

- AFL devices often require only one treatment but reappraisal of photodamage, rhytides, or scarring can be performed at the 6- to 12-month postoperative period and, if necessary, a second AFL treatment can be performed if clinically warranted. Settings for a commonly used AFL (Fraxel re:pair) range from 20 to 100 mJ with treatment densities of 600 to 1600 MTZ/cm². The Lumenis system (Total Fx) has 2 heads with variable energies (Deep FX: 15–25 mJ, Active FX: 80–125 mJ) and densities (Deep FX: 10%–15%, Active RX: 1%–3%) depending on the severity of scarring.

- Optimal treatment settings vary depending on the laser used and the severity of each individual's scarring. There is evidence that suggests patient satisfaction and clinical results improve with increasing fluences. Increased postoperative adverse events (pain, erythema, dyspigmentation) are more often observed when higher treatment densities are selected.

- Patients who receive NAFL treatment should use a mild cleanser and moisturizer several times daily for the first few days after each treatment session (or as long as bronzing/xerosis is apparent). Sun exposure should be avoided during this time.

- Postoperative erythema resolves spontaneously, but its intensity and duration may be reduced by immediate treatment with a 590-nm wavelength light-emitting diode (LED) array.

- Those who receive treatment with an AFL must undergo open-wound or closed-wound care as previously described for the first several postoperative days. Thereafter, patients can slowly resume the use of their regular skin-care products.

- Adverse events reported with fractional lasers:

Mild	Moderate	Severe
Prolonged erythema	Infection	Hypertrophic scarring
Acne and milia	Pigmentary alteration	Ectropion formation
Delayed purpura	Anesthesia toxicity	Disseminated infection
Superficial erosions	Eruptive keratoacanthomas	
Contact dermatitis		
Recall phenomenon		

The optimal settings will vary depending on the laser used and the severity and type of scarring present. Higher energy settings may result in improved clinical efficacy, but are also associated with increased adverse events (pain, erythema, postoperative dyspigmentation).[109,110] Patients who receive NAFL treatment should use a mild cleanser and moisturizer several times daily for

Table 1
Handling side effects and complications of ablative and fractional skin resurfacing

Side Effect/Complication	When to Look for It	Treatment
Prolonged erythema	1 month+	• Avoid use of irritating topicals • Apply mild corticosteroid • LED photomodulation
Milia/acne exacerbation	1 month+	• Discontinue occlusive dressings/ointments • Physical extraction of milia • Oral antibiotics for acne
Contact/allergic dermatitis	Any time	• Discontinue allergen/irritant • Topical/oral corticosteroid • Oral antihistamine
Infection	1–14 days	• Take appropriate cultures • Oral antibacterial/antiviral • Topical wound care
Hyperpigmentation	1 month+	• Topical lighteners • Mild chemical peels • Sunscreen
Hypopigmentation	6 months+	• Excimer laser • Topical photochemotherapy
Hypertrophic scar	1 month+	• Potent topical corticosteroid • Pulsed dye laser
Ectropion	1 month+	• Surgical correction

the first few days after each treatment session (or as long as bronzing/xerosis is apparent). Sun exposure should be avoided during this time. Postoperative erythema resolves spontaneously but its intensity and duration may be reduced by immediate treatment with a 590-nm wavelength LED array.[111] On the other hand, those who receive treatment with an AFL must undergo open-wound or closed-wound care as previously described for the first several postoperative days. Thereafter, patients can slowly resume the use of their regular skin-care products.

Patients who undergo NAFL sessions on a monthly basis show progressive improvement with each successive treatment. Skin resurfacing with AFL does not require as many sessions to observe clinical improvement. Most patients require only 1 or 2 AFL treatments at 6- to 12-months intervals. It is has been theorized that the enhanced clinical effects of AFLs are related to their ability to penetrate more deeply into the skin compared with fully ablative lasers and NAFLs, and also to a prolonged wound remodeling response of several months' duration.

Fractional skin resurfacing is associated with a relatively low complication rate.[109,110] Most untoward events of NAFL treatment are mild and transient, including erythema, periocular edema, xerosis, and slight darkening of the skin (bronzing) during desquamation of the microscopic epidermal necrotic debris.[109] The most commonly encountered adverse events reported are acneiform and herpetic eruptions in fewer than 2% of patients. Postinflammatory hyperpigmentation may also occur, particularly in patients with darker skin phototypes.[89] Intense erythema, serosanguinous drainage, and crusting are typical for 5 to 7 days after AFL treatment (compared with 2 to 3 days with NAFL).[110] Caution must be advised when treating skin in areas that are thin or devoid of pilosebaceous units. Although rare, hypertrophic scarring of the neck, chest, and periocular regions has been reported with AFLs,[112,113] so overly aggressive treatment settings should be avoided in these sensitive anatomic sites. To date, permanent pigmentary alteration has not been reported. Other exceedingly rare adverse events such as eruptive keratoacanthomas and recall phenomenon also have been reported.[114,115] **Table 1** presents fractional laser side effects and complications.

SUMMARY

Cutaneous injuries that result in scar tissue formation are a result of overly exuberant wound healing. Scars are relatively common and lead patients to seek treatment for cosmetic or functional improvement. At present, the many medical treatments that are available for these maladies often prove inadequate or inconvenient. It is precisely for these

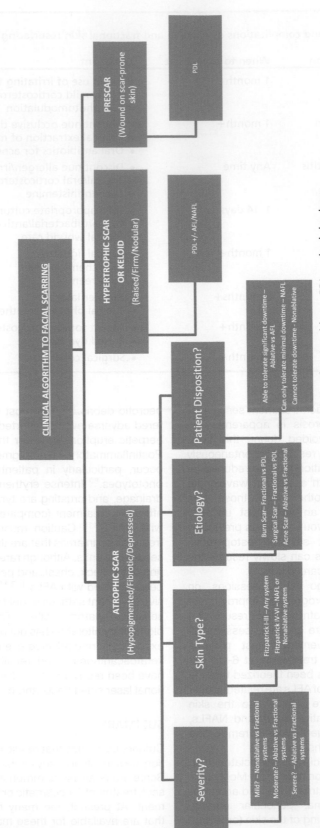

Fig. 5. Clinical algorithm to facial scarring. AFL, ablative fractional laser; NAFL, nonablative fractional laser; PDL, pulsed dye laser.

reasons that laser therapy has been investigated for improvement of scars and ulcerations.

There are several laser systems available that permit successful treatment of various types of scars, and **Fig. 5** displays the laser scar revision treatment algorithm. The 585-nm PDL remains the gold standard for laser treatment of hypertrophic scars and keloids. In addition, the PDL has been shown to lead to more rapid healing of pre-scars. Atrophic scars may best be treated with ablative and fractionally ablative and nonablative laser systems, depending on the specific circumstances of each patient. Nonablative systems, although less clinically efficacious, may be used in patients desiring a treatment with reduced post-operative recovery. Laser scar revision is optimized when individual patient and scar characteristics are thoroughly evaluated to determine the best course of treatment and, more importantly, to determine whether the patient and physician share realistic expectations and treatment goals.

REFERENCES

1. Levine E, Degutis L, Pruzinsky T, et al. Quality of life and facial trauma: psychological and body image effects. Ann Plast Surg 2005;54:502–10.

2. Robert R, Meyer W, Bishop S, et al. Disfiguring burn scars and adolescent self-esteem. Burns 1999;25:581–5.

3. Tebble NJ, Adams R, Thomas DW, et al. Anxiety and self-consciousness in patients with facial lacerations one week and six months later. Br J Oral Maxillofac Surg 2006;44:520–5.

4. Bell L, McAdams T, Morgan R, et al. Pruritus in burns: a descriptive study. J Burn Care Rehabil 1988;9:305–11.

5. Young VL, Hutchison J. Insights into patient and clinician concerns about scar appearance: semi-quantitative structured surveys. Plast Reconstr Surg 2009;124:256–65.

6. Rumsey N, Clarke A, White P. Exploring the psychosocial concerns of outpatients with disfiguring conditions. J Wound Care 2003;12:247–52.

7. Brown BC, McKenna SP, Siddhi K, et al. The hidden cost of skin scars: quality of life after skin scarring. J Plast Reconstr Aesthet Surg 2008;61:1049–58.

8. Urioste SS, Arndt KA, Dover JS. Keloids and hypertrophic scars: review and treatment strategies. Semin Cutan Med Surg 1999;18:159–71.

9. Monaco JL, Lawrence WT. Acute wound healing: an overview. Clin Plast Surg 2003;30:1–12.

10. Reish RG, Eriksson E. Scars: a review of emerging and currently available therapies. Plast Reconstr Surg 2008;122:1068–78.

11. Alster TS, Tanzi EL. Hypertrophic scars and keloids: etiology and management. Am J Clin Dermatol 2003;4:235–43.

12. Ferguson MWJ, Duncan J, Bond J, et al. Prophylactic administration of avotermin for improvement of skin scarring: three double-blind placebo-controlled phase I/II studies. Lancet 2009;373:1264–74.

13. Wu WS, Wang FS, Yang KD, et al. Dexamethasone induction of keloid regression through effective suppression of VEGF expression and keloid fibroblast proliferation. J Invest Dermatol 2006;126:1264–71.

14. Mallick KS, Hajek AS, Parrish RK. Fluorouracil (5-FU) and cytarabine (ara-C) inhibition of corneal epithelial cell and conjunctival fibroblast proliferation. Arch Ophthalmol 1985;103:1398–402.

15. Hendricks T, Martens MF, Huyben CM, et al. Inhibition of basal and TGF beta-induced fibroblast collagen synthesis by antineoplastic agents: implications for wound healing. Br J Cancer 1993;67:545–50.

16. Asilian A, Darougheh A, Shariati F. New combination of triamcinolone, 5-fluorouracil, and pulsed-dye laser for treatment of keloid and hypertrophic scars. Dermatol Surg 2006;32:907–15.

17. Fitzpatrick RE. Treatment of inflamed hypertrophic scars using intralesional 5-FU. Dermatol Surg 1999;25:224–32.

18. Ragoowansi R, Cornes PG, Moss AL, et al. Treatment of keloids by surgical excision and immediate postoperative single-fraction radiotherapy. Plast Reconstr Surg 2003;111:1853–9.

19. Anderson RR, Parrish JA. Selective photothermolysis: precise microsurgery by selective absorption of pulsed radiation. Science 1983;22:524–7.

20. Alster TS, Kurban AK, Grove GL, et al. Alteration of argon laser-induced scars by the pulsed dye laser. Lasers Surg Med 1993;13:368–73.

21. Powers PS, Sarkar S, Goldgof DB, et al. Scar assessment: current problems and future solutions. J Burn Care Rehabil 1999;20:54–9.

22. Yeong EK, Mann R, Engrav LH, et al. Improved burn scar assessment with use of a new scar-rating scale. J Burn Care Rehabil 1997;18:353–5.

23. Nedelec B, Shankowsky HA, Tredget EE. Rating the resolving hypertrophic scar: comparison of the Vancouver scar scale and scar volume. J Burn Care Rehabil 2000;21:205–12.

24. Draaijers LJ, Templeman FRH, Botman YAM, et al. The patient and observer scar assessment scale: a reliable and feasible tool for scar evaluation. Plast Reconstr Surg 2004;113:1960–5.

25. Idriss N, Maibach HI. Scar assessment scales: a dermatologic overview. Skin Res Technol 2009;15:1–5.

26. Jacob CI, Dover JS, Kaminer MS. Acne scarring: a classification system and review of treatment options. J Am Acad Dermatol 2001;45:109–17.

27. McCraw JB, McCraw JA, McMellin A, et al. Prevention of unfavorable scars using early pulsed dye laser treatments: a preliminary report. Ann Plast Surg 1999;42:7–14.

28. Bowes LE, Alster TS. Treatment of facial scarring and ulceration resulting from acne excoriée with 585-nm pulsed dye laser irradiation and cognitive psychotherapy. Dermatol Surg 2004;30:934–8.

29. Nouri K, Jimenez GP, Harrison-Balestra C, et al. 585-nm pulsed dye laser in the treatment of surgical scars starting on the suture removal day. Dermatol Surg 2003;29:65–73.

30. Pinheiro AL, Pozza DH, Oliveira MG, et al. Polarized light (400–2000 nm) and non-ablative laser (685 nm): a description of the wound healing process using immunohistochemistry analysis. Photomed Laser Surg 2005;23:485–92.

31. Bouzari N, Davis SC, Nouri K. Laser treatment of keloids and hypertrophic scars. Int J Dermatol 2007;46:80–8.

32. Alster TS, Zaulyanov-Scanlon L. Laser scar revision: a review. Dermatol Surg 2007;33:131–40.

33. Castro DJ, Abergel RP, Meeker C, et al. Effects of the Nd:YAG laser on DNA synthesis and collagen production in human skin fibroblast cultures. Ann Plast Surg 1983;11:214–22.

34. Abergel RP, Meeker CA, Lam TS, et al. Control of connective tissue metabolism by lasers: recent developments and future prospects. J Am Acad Dermatol 1984;11:1142–50.

35. Henderson DL, Cromwell TA, Mes LG. Argon and carbon dioxide laser treatment of hypertrophic and keloid scars. Lasers Surg Med 1984;3:271.

36. Abergel RP, Dwyer RM, Meeker CA, et al. Laser treatment of keloids: a clinical trial and an in vitro study with Nd:YAG laser. Lasers Surg Med 1984;4:291–5.

37. Alster TS, Williams CM. Improvement of keloid sternotomy scars by the 585 nm pulsed dye laser: a controlled study. Lancet 1995;345:1198–200.

38. Alster TS. Improvement of erythematous and hypertrophic scars by the 585 nm flashlamp-pumped pulsed dye laser. Ann Plast Surg 1994;32(2):186–90.

39. Alster TS, Nanni CA. Pulsed dye laser treatment of hypertrophic burn scars. Plast Reconstr Surg 1998;102:2190–5.

40. Alster TS, McMeekin TO. Improvement of facial acne scars by the 585nm flashlamp-pumped pulsed dye laser. J Am Acad Dermatol 1996;35:79–81.

41. Alster TS. Laser treatment of scars and striae. In: Alster TS, editor. Manual of cutaneous laser techniques. Philadelphia: Lippincott- Raven; 2000. p. 89–107.

42. Kuo YR, Jeng SF, Wang FS, et al. Flashlamp pulsed dye laser (PDL) suppression of keloid proliferation through down-regulation of TGF-beta1 expression and extracellular matrix expression. Lasers Surg Med 2004;34:104–8.

43. Reiken SR, Wolfort SF, Berthiamume F, et al. Control of hypertrophic scar growth using selective photothermolysis. Lasers Surg Med 1997;21:7–12.

44. Manuskiatti W, Wanitphakdeedecha R, Fitzpatrick RE. Effect of pulse width of a 595-nm flashlamp-pumped pulsed dye laser on the treatment response of keloidal and hypertrophic sternotomy scars. Dermatol Surg 2007;33:152–61.

45. Shah S, Alster TS. Laser treatment of dark skin: an updated review. Am J Clin Dermatol 2010;11:1–10.

46. Bhatt N, Alster TS. Laser surgery in dark skin. Dermatol Surg 2008;34:184–95.

47. Alster TS. Laser scar revision: comparison of pulsed dye laser with and without intralesional corticosteroids. Dermatol Surg 2002;29:25–9.

48. Manuskiatti W, Fitzpatrick RE. Treatment response of keloidal and hypertrophic sternotomy scars: comparison among intralesional corticosteroid, 5-fluorouracil, and 585-nm flashlamp-pumped pulsed-dye laser treatments. Arch Dermatol 2002;138:1149–55.

49. Hermanns JF, Petit L, Hermanns LT, et al. Analytic quantification of phototype-related regional skin complexion. Skin Res Technol 2001;7:168–71.

50. Fiskerstrand EJ, Svaasand LO, Volden G. Pigmentary changes after pulsed dye laser treatment in 125 northern European patients with port wine stains. Br J Dermatol 1998;138(3):477–9.

51. Bellew SG, Weiss MA, Weiss RA. Comparison of intense pulsed light to 585-nm long-pulsed pulsed dye laser for treatment of hypertrophic surgical scars: a pilot study. J Drugs Dermatol 2005;4:448–52.

52. Bowes LE, Nouri K, Berman B, et al. Treatment of pigmented hypertrophic scars with the 585nm pulsed dye laser and the 532 nm frequency-doubled Nd:YAG laser in the Q-switched and variable pulse modes: a comparative study. Dermatol Surg 2002;28:714–9.

53. Apfelberg DB, Maser MR, White DN, et al. Failure of carbon dioxide laser excision of keloids. Lasers Surg Med 1989;9:382–8.

54. Tanzi EL, Wanitphakdeedecha R, Alster TS. Fraxel laser indications and long-term follow-up. Aesthet Surg J 2008;28:61–4.

55. Alster TS. Cutaneous resurfacing with CO_2 and erbium: YAG laser: preoperative, intraoperative, and postoperative considerations. Plast Reconstr Surg 1999;103:619–32.

56. Alster TS, Tanzi EL. Laser skin resurfacing: ablative and nonablative. In: Robinson J, Sengelman R, Siegel DM, et al, editors. Surgery of the skin. Philadelphia: Elsevier; 2005. p. 611–24.

57. Alster TS, West TB. Resurfacing atrophic facial scars with a high energy, pulsed carbon dioxide laser. Dermatol Surg 1996;22:151–5.

58. Walia S, Alster TS. Prolonged clinical and histological effects from CO_2 laser resurfacing of atrophic scars. Dermatol Surg 1999;25:926–30.

59. Tanzi EL, Alster TS. Treatment of atrophic facial acne scars with a dual-mode Er: YAG laser. Dermatol Surg 2002;28:551–5.

60. Alster TS, Nanni CA, Williams CM. Comparison of four carbon dioxide resurfacing lasers: a clinical and histopathologic evaluation. Dermatol Surg 1999;25:153–9.

61. Alster TS, Kauvar AN, Geronemus RG. Histology of high-energy pulsed CO_2 laser resurfacing. Semin Cutan Med Surg 1996;15:189–93.

62. Ross EV, Grossman MC, Duke D, et al. Long-term results after CO_2 laser skin resurfacing: a comparison of scanned and pulsed systems. J Am Acad Dermatol 1997;37:709–18.

63. Green D, Egbert BM, Utley DS, et al. In vivo model of histologic changes after treatment with the super-pulsed CO_2 laser, erbium: YAG laser, and blended lasers: a 4- to 6-month prospective histologic and clinical study. Lasers Surg Med 2000;27:362–72.

64. Fitzpatrick RE, Tope WD, Goldman MP, et al. Pulsed carbon dioxide laser, trichloroacetic acid, Baker-Gordon phenol, and dermabrasion: a comparative clinical and histologic study of cutaneous resurfacing in a porcine model. Arch Dermatol 1996;132:469–71.

65. Fitzpatrick RE, Smith SR, Sriprachya-Anunt S. Depth of vaporization and the effect of pulse stacking with a high-energy, pulsed CO_2 laser. J Am Acad Dermatol 1999;40:615–22.

66. Fitzpatrick RE, Rostan EF, Marchell N. Collagen tightening induced by carbon dioxide laser versus erbium:YAG laser. Lasers Surg Med 2000;27:395–403.

67. Katz BE, MacFarlane DF. Atypical facial scarring after isotretinoin therapy in a patient with a previous dermabrasion. J Am Acad Dermatol 1994;30:852–3.

68. Nanni CA, Alster TS. Complications of CO_2 laser resurfacing: an evaluation of 500 patients. Dermatol Surg 1998;24:315–20.

69. Horton S, Alster TS. Preoperative and postoperative considerations for cutaneous laser resurfacing. Cutis 1999;64:399–406.

70. Alster TS, Lupton JR. Prevention and treatment of side effects and complications of cutaneous laser resurfacing. Plast Reconstr Surg 2002;109:308–16.

71. Walia S, Alster TS. Cutaneous CO_2 laser resurfacing infection rate with and without prophylactic antibiotics. Dermatol Surg 1999;25:857–61.

72. Alster TS, Nanni CA. Famciclovir prophylaxis of herpes simplex virus reactivation after cutaneous laser resurfacing. Dermatol Surg 1997;25:242–6.

73. Beeson WH, Rachel JD. Valacyclovir prophylaxis for herpes simplex virus infection or infection recurrence following laser skin resurfacing. Dermatol Surg 2002;28:331–6.

74. Fisher AA. Lasers and allergic contact dermatitis to topical antibiotics, with particular reference to bacitracin. Cutis 1996;58:252–4.

75. Tanzi EL, Alster TS. Comparison of a 1450 nm diode laser and a 1320 nm Nd:YAG laser in the treatment of atrophic facial scars: a prospective clinical and histological study. Dermatol Surg 2004;30:152–7.

76. Rogachefsky AS, Hussain M, Goldberg DJ. Atrophic and mixed pattern of acne scars with a 1320 nm Nd:YAG laser. Dermatol Surg 2003;29:904–8.

77. Friedman PM, Jih MH, Skover GR, et al. Treatment of atrophic facial acne scars with the 1064-nm Q-switched Nd:YAG laser. Arch Dermatol 2004;140:1337–41.

78. Friedman PM, Skover GR, Payonik G, et al. 3D in-vivo optical skin imaging for topographical quantitative assessment of non-ablative laser technology. Dermatol Surg 2002;28:199–204.

79. Sobanko JF, Alster TS. Laser skin resurfacing of rhytides and scars. In: Spiegel J, editor. Office based facial plastic surgery, in press.

80. Manstein D, Herron GS, Sink RK, et al. Fractional photothermolysis: a new concept for cutaneous remodeling using microscopic patterns of thermal injury. Lasers Surg Med 2004;34:426–38.

81. Laubach HJ, Tannous Z, Anderson RR, et al. Skin responses to fractional photothermolysis. Lasers Surg Med 2006;38:142–9.

82. Walgrave S, Zelickson B, Childs J, et al. Pilot investigation of the correlation between histological and clinical effects of infrared fractional resurfacing lasers. Dermatol Surg 2008;34:1443–53.

83. Geronemus R. Fractional photothermolysis: current and future applications. Lasers Surg Med 2006;38:169–76.

84. Alster TS, Tanzi EL, Lazarus E. The use of fractional laser photothermolysis for the treatment of atrophic scars. Dermatol Surg 2007;33:295–9.

85. Taub AF. Fractionated delivery systems for difficult to treat clinical applications: acne scarring, melasma, atrophic scarring, striae distensae, and deep rhytides. J Drugs Dermatol 2007;6:1120–8.

86. Chrastil B, Glaich AS, Goldberg LH, et al. Second-generation 1,550-nm fractional photothermolysis for the treatment of acne scars. Dermatol Surg 2008;34:1327–32.

87. Hu S, Chen MC, Lee MC, et al. Fractional resurfacing for the treatment of atrophic facial acne scars in Asian skin. Dermatol Surg 2009;35:826–32.

88. Cho SB, Le JH, Choi MJ, et al. Efficacy of the fractional photothermolysis system with dynamic operating mode on acne scars and enlarged pores. Dermatol Surg 2009;35:108–14.

89. Mahmoud BH, Srivastava D, Janiga JJ, et al. Safety and efficacy of erbium-doped yttrium aluminum garnet fractionated laser for treatment of acne

scars in type IV to VI skin. Dermatol Surg 2010;36: 602–9.

90. Vasily DB, Cerino ME, Ziselman EM, et al. Non-ablative fractional resurfacing of surgical and post-traumatic scars. J Drugs Dermatol 2009;8: 998–1005.

91. Haedersdal M, Morean KER, Beyer DM, et al. Fractional nonablative 1540 nm laser resurfacing for thermal burn scars: a randomized controlled trial. Lasers Surg Med 2009;41:189–95.

92. Tierney EP, Kouba DJ, Hanke CW. Review of fractional photothermolysis: treatment indications and efficacy. Dermatol Surg 2009;35:1445–61.

93. Kunishige JH, Katz TM, Goldberg LH, et al. Fractional photothermolysis for the treatment of surgical scars. Dermatol Surg 2010;36:538–41.

94. Manstein D, Zurakowski D, Thongsima S, et al. The effects of multiple passes on the epidermal thermal damage pattern in nonablative fractional resurfacing. Lasers Surg Med 2009;41:149–53.

95. Thongsima S, Zurakowski D, Manstein D. Histological comparison of two different fractional photothermolysis devices operating at 1,550nm. Lasers Surg Med 2010;42:32–7.

96. Hantash BM, Bedi VP, Kapadia B, et al. In vivo histological evaluation of a novel ablative fractional resurfacing device. Lasers Surg Med 2007;39: 96–107.

97. Saluja R, Khoury J, Detwiler SP, et al. Histologic and clinical response to varying density settings with a fractionally scanned carbon dioxide laser. J Drugs Dermatol 2009;8:17–20.

98. Prignano F, Campolmi P, Bonan P, et al. Fractional CO_2 laser: a novel therapeutic device upon photomodulation of tissue remodeling and cytokine pathway of tissue repair. Dermatol Ther 2009;22:S8–15.

99. Waibel J, Beer K, Narurkar V, et al. Preliminary observations on fractional ablative resurfacing devices: clinical impressions. J Drugs Dermatol 2009;8:481–5.

100. Chappas AM, Brightman L, Sukal S, et al. Successful treatment of acneiform scarring with CO_2 ablative fractional resurfacing. Lasers Surg Med 2008; 40:381–6.

101. Cho SB, Lee SJ, Kang JM, et al. The efficacy and safety of 10,600-nm carbon dioxide fractional laser for acne scars in Asian patients. Dermatol Surg 2009;35:1955–61.

102. Walgrave SE, Ortiz AE, MacFalls HT, et al. Evaluation of a novel fractional resurfacing device for the treatment of acne scarring. Lasers Surg Med 2009; 41:122–7.

103. Gotkin RH, Sarnoff DS, Cannarozzo G et al. Ablative skin resurfacing with a novel microablative CO_2 laser. J Drugs Dermatol 1009;8:138–144.

104. Kim S, Cho KH. Clinical trial of dual treatment with an ablative fractional laser and a nonablative laser for the treatment of acne scars in Asian patients. Dermatol Surg 2009;35:1089–98.

105. Ortiz AE, Tremaine AM, Zachary CB. Long-term efficacy of a fractional resurfacing device. Lasers Surg Med 2010;42:168–70.

106. Manuskiatti W, Triwongwaranat D, Varothai S, et al. Efficacy and safety of a carbon-dioxide ablative fractional resurfacing device for treatment of atrophic acne scars in Asians. J Am Acad Dermatol 2010;63:274–83.

107. Weiss ET, Chapas A, Brightman L, et al. Successful treatment of atrophic postoperative and traumatic scarring with carbon dioxide ablative fractional resurfacing. Arch Dermatol 2010;146:133–40.

108. Waibel J, Beer K. Ablative fractional laser resurfacing for the treatment of a third-degree burn. J Drugs Dermatol 2009;8:294–7.

109. Graber EM, Tanzi EL, Alster TS. Side effects and complications of fractional laser photothermolysis: experience with 961 treatments. Dermatol Surg 2008;34:301–7.

110. Metelitsa AI, Alster TS. Fractionated laser skin resurfacing treatment complications: a review. Dermatol Surg 2010;36:299–306.

111. Alster TS, Wanitphakdeedecha R. Improvement of post-fractional laser erythema with light-emitting diode photomodulation. Dermatol Surg 2009;35: 813–5.

112. Avram MM, Tope WD, Yu T, et al. Hypertrophic scarring of the neck following ablative fractional carbon dioxide laser resurfacing. Lasers Surg Med 2009;41:185–8.

113. Fife DJ, Fitzpatrick RE, Zachary CB. Complications of fractional CO_2 laser resurfacing: four cases. Lasers Surg Med 2009;41:179–84.

114. Mamelak AJ, Goldberg LH, Marquez D, et al. Eruptive keratoacanthomas on the legs after fractional photothermolysis: report of two cases. Dermatol Surg 2009;35:513–8.

115. Foster KW, Fincher EF, Moy RL. Heat-induced "recall" of treatment zone erythema following fractional resurfacing with a combination laser (1320 nm/1440 nm). Arch Dermatol 2008;144:1398–9.

Use of Lasers in Acute Management of Surgical and Traumatic Incisions on the Face

Sepehr Oliaei, MD[a,b], J. Stuart Nelson, MD, PhD[a],
Richard Fitzpatrick, MD[c], Brian J. Wong, MD, PhD[a,b,*]

KEYWORDS

- Traumatic scars • Laser scar revision • Acute
- Soft tissue injury • Pulsed dye laser
- Carbon dioxide • Fractional laser

This article discusses use of laser technologies in acute management of soft tissue injuries in surgical incisions and trauma. To minimize scar formation, current standard of care in acute management of surgical incisions includes irrigation and cleansing, multilayered, tension-free closure with precise approximation and eversion of wound edges, judicious use of suture material, use of postoperative moisture barrier or dressing, and early removal of surgical sutures. Traumatic soft tissue injury involving the skin can be more challenging to manage acutely due to frequent presence of crushed, macerated, or otherwise devitalized tissues. Additional steps are often warranted in that setting including removal of foreign bodies, copious irrigation of the wound, removal of clearly devitalized tissues, and use of antibiotics to cover polymicrobial flora. Despite these measures, poor cosmetic outcome is frequent after surgical procedures and traumatic skin injuries.

Numerous adjunctive measures have been proposed to optimize wound healing and obviate the need for operative scar revision, many of which are discussed in this volume. These include use of steroids, post-treatment dressings, avoidance of sunlight, dermabrasion, and laser treatment. In classic dermabrasion, mechanical debridement of the superficial papillary dermis leads to re-epithelialization via the adnexal structures, resulting in improved texture and color of the skin. This is an excellent method for smoothing an irregular surface or correcting pigmentary discrepancy between adjacent skin edges, which alters how light creates shadows across the surface. Dermabrasion is recommended 6 to 8 weeks after injury/surgical procedure. More substantial improvements are reported during this period, as the immature scar is still undergoing remodeling, rather than during the mature phase.[1] Proposed mechanism of action for this modality has been described by Harmon and colleagues[2] as reorganization of connective tissue ultrastructure and epithelial cell–cell interactions with an increase in collagen bundle density and size with a tendency

Financial Disclosures: None.
Conflicts of Interest: None.
[a] Beckman Laser Institute and Medical Clinic, University Of California Irvine, 1002 Health Sciences Road, Irvine, CA 92612, USA
[b] Division of Facial Plastic Surgery, Department of Otolaryngology-Head and Neck Surgery, University of California Irvine, 101 The City Drive South, Building 56, Suite 500, Orange, CA 92868, USA
[c] Cosmetic Laser Dermatology, 9339 Genesee Avenue 300, San Diego, CA 92121, USA
* Corresponding author. Division of Facial Plastic Surgery, Department of Otolaryngology-Head and Neck Surgery, University of California Irvine, 101 The City Drive South, Building 56, Suite 500, Orange, CA 92868.
E-mail address: bjwong@uci.edu

Facial Plast Surg Clin N Am 19 (2011) 543–550
doi:10.1016/j.fsc.2011.06.007

toward unidirectional orientation of fibers parallel to the epidermal surface. Although excellent outcomes have been described with this technique, it does require a fair level of operator experience and learning curve for manual control of the depth of dermabrasion and feathering of the edges. Additionally, this technique can be complicated with excessive bleeding and tearing of tissues at the treatment margin. Laser scar revision is a competing technology that has gained increasing popularity due to the potential for excellent hemostasis, ease of use, and precise control over depth of penetration and extent of treatment.

Since the introduction of laser skin resurfacing for aesthetic surgery in the mid-1990s, the technology has worked its way into broad use in scar revision. Laser and optical methods for management of acute injury have very vital roles in postsurgical and traumatic wound therapeutic outcome. With advances in this technology a clinician may arrive at a crossroads in the decision to treat a scar with surgical revision versus dermabrasion or various laser technologies. The authors present and review their experience herein to help with this decision-making process in the acute setting. This article discusses indications and strengths of available optical modalities with a focus on acute and subacute skin injuries. The discussion is practically oriented and structured around the specific applications of each technology.

ACUTE COSMETIC MANAGEMENT OF SURGICAL WOUNDS

Scars can be disfiguring, aesthetically unacceptable, and cause pruritis, tenderness, pain, sleep disturbance, anxiety, and depression in postsurgical patients. Regardless of the specific strategy for treatment, current optical technologies offer the reconstructive surgeon valuable tools to lessen the psychological burden of undergoing surgery by optimizing the cosmetic outcome in a noninvasive or minimally invasive form. Availability of these tools can lead to higher levels of patient satisfaction after surgery.

For purposes of this discussion, a surgical incision is defined as an incision that is closed per standard of care as discussed previously with optimal postsurgical care and without perioperative wound complications. Ideal post-surgical scar is flat, flexible and indiscernible from surrounding skin in terms of color and texture. Despite optimal wound closure and postoperative care, aberrant fibroblast response can lead to hypertrophic or keloid scars, and aberrant angiogenesis may lead to telangiectasias or a hyperemic scar. Imperfect surgical closure or poor postoperative

management can lead to poor outcomes with step-offs, depressions, suture marks, dyspigmentation, or broad hypertrophic scars due to wound tension or distal flap vascular compromise and tissue necrosis. Abnormal collagen deposition has been demonstrated histologically in hypertrophic scars with elevated levels of collagen 3[3] Traditionally improved via mechanical dermabrasion, the current arsenal for optimization of surgical wounds includes various optical technologies such as conventional ablative laser resurfacing and nonablative laser treatment, as well as fractionated and pulsed laser technologies. Acute optimization of wound healing can start immediately after the completion of surgery as in laser-assisted scar healing (LASH)[4] or after removal of sutures within 1 week postoperatively, or it may focus on treatment of maturing scar several weeks to months after surgery.

ACUTE COSMETIC MANAGEMENT OF TRAUMATIC WOUNDS

Some injuries such as uncomplicated linear lacerations are indistinguishable from surgical incisions. The challenge with traumatic skin injuries lies in irregular borders, high tension, macerated tissue, and tissue loss. More often than not, traumatic lacerations involve nonlinear or stellate disruption of the epidermis that is not at right angle to the skin surface. Traumatic abrasions can harbor foreign bodies, which if not adequately debrided, can lead to traumatic tattooing. Presence of tissue edema, hematoma, and loss of tissue can force a high-tension closure, which can lead to broad hypertrophic scarring. Risk of infection is compounded by inadequate cleansing and irrigation of tissues and lack of proper antibiotic coverage after repair. Devitalized, necrosed skin edges and infected wounds can lead to severe atrophic or hypertrophic scars and extremely poor cosmetic outcomes. Use of copious irrigation and antibiotic coverage for gram-positive skin flora with first- or second-generation cephalosporins or clindamycin should be considered in these patients. In the case of an animal or human bite or other gross contaminations of the wound, appropriate adjustments to the antibiotic coverage must be made.

Due to the specific patient population as well as the treatment setting, poor follow-up is often an issue with these patients, leading to improper postoperative care such as suture retention or delay in diagnosis of wound infection. Use of rapidly absorbing suture material where available and appropriate is therefore advised in traumatic skin closure, particularly in those whose attention to follow-up is uncertain. Delayed presentation to the surgeon can also be an issue in this population, as the patient is often acutely managed by an emergency room physician, family doctor, physician assistant, or a general surgeon as opposed to a specialist with reconstructive surgical expertise. Intervention should occur as early as possible following presentation to prevent progression in the direction of an undesirable mature scar that may require surgical revision.

OPTICAL MANAGEMENT OF ACUTE SURGICAL AND TRAUMATIC WOUNDS

This discussion encompasses conventional ablative resurfacing lasers, pulsed dye laser (PDL), and fractionated lasers for acute cosmetic optimization of surgical and traumatic wounds.

Ablative Laser Resurfacing

Traditional laser resurfacing is a technique that is commonly accomplished via ablative devices such as conventional carbon dioxide (CO_2) or Erbium:YAG lasers. Mechanism of action is similar to using a mechanical dermabrader with the potential to modulate wound healing through thermal effects of laser and trigger the same regenerative mechanisms as when these devices are used for classic facial resurfacing. Tissue removal by laser is a function of treatment parameters, tissue optical properties, and tissue thermal properties. Histologically, laser-treated skin shows a subepidermal dermal repair zone consisting of compact new collagen fibers overlying collagen with evidence of solar elastosis.[5] Because it is possible to achieve discrete, measurable incremental amounts of tissue removal with each pulse, only a modest level of skill is required for achieving optimal results.

CO_2

The CO_2 laser is the work horse of cosmetic dermatology and the model to which all optical therapies are compared. Despite nearly 20 years of use, CO_2 laser skin resurfacing remains very valuable due to the capacity to remove bulk amounts of tissue in a bloodless fashion, and correct iatrogenic contour irregularities. Differences of outcomes between CO_2 and dermabrasion remain incompletely understood.[6,7] However, due to decreasing technology associated costs, CO_2 laser resurfacing has slowly gained popularity. CO_2 laser is emitted at wavelengths ranging from 9400 to 10,600 nm, and it is preferentially absorbed by water (its principal chromophore), leading to superficial ablation of tissue by vaporization. Although the majority of the energy is absorbed by the first 20 to 30 µm of the skin, the zone of thermal damage can be as

much as 1 mm deep.[8] This is in part responsible for the persistent erythema experienced by patients that can continue for 6 months or longer after CO_2 laser treatment, but it may also contribute to enhanced collagen remodeling. Timing of the treatment is typically the same as mechanical dermabrasion, optimally performed 4 to 8 weeks after the initial injury. The ideal application of this laser is for induction of contour changes and collagen remodeling in elevated scars.

Erbium:YAG Laser

Introduced to dermatology in the mid-1990s, the Erbium:YAG laser also removes tissue, but the penetration depth of the wavelength (2936 nm) is shallow, as is the corresponding depth of thermal injury. Light from this laser is absorbed 12 to 18 times more efficiently by water compared with the CO_2 laser. However, the more superficial depth of penetration and surrounding tissue injury lead to decreased induction of collagen remodeling and contraction.[9] Due to poor coagulative properties, hemostasis can also be a problem with this modality, particularly if extensive tissue needs to be removed. Application of this laser is for generating subtle contour changes in depressed and atrophic scars. Additionally, the Erbium:YAG laser may be used in cases where thermal injury is undesirable (such as a known keloid former).

PDL

PDL relies upon concept of selective photothermolysis.[10] The 585 to 595 nm wavelengths are preferentially absorbed by hemoglobin, although epidermal melanin absorption can be of concern in patients with darker skin phototypes. This selectivity makes this technology ideal for in the treatment of vascular lesions skin lesions such as telangiectasia, port wine stains, and hemangiomas. During scar treatment, PDL destroys the blood supply to the wound edge at the level of dermal microvasculature, inhibiting the formation of scars. The angiolytic mechanism of action has been disputed by some authors.[11] Alternatively, changes in cell cycle distribution of fibroblasts in keloid scars has been proposed recently as a mechanism of action of PDL treatment in keloid scars.[12]

Properties of this laser make it suitable for treatment of red, hyperemic, hypertrophic scars, and keloids (**Figs. 1–3**). PDL improves color, texture, and pliability of scars by reducing pigmentation, vascularity, and bulk of scar tissue.[13] Because it spares the epidermal and dermal tissues, treatment can be repeated at 6- to 8-week intervals with significantly reduced downtime and erythema

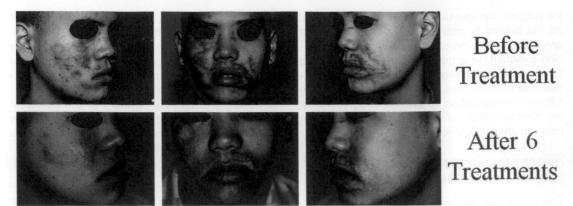

Before Treatment

After 6 Treatments

Fig. 1. Hypervascular scar treated using the pulsed dye laser. Top: before treatment. Bottom: after treatment.

compared with conventional CO_2 laser resurfacing. Due to competitive absorption of the emitted energy by melanin, darker toned individuals (Fitzpatrick IV-V) may not be suitable candidates for this treatment due to risk of dyspigmentation.[14] The authors' parameters for PDL wound optimization are listed in **Table 1**.

Fractional Photothermolysis

Fractional photothermolysis, first introduced by Manstein and colleagues[15] in 2004, is the latest in the available phototherapeutics for scars. Fractionation refers to a technology in which thousands of pinpoint laser beams are directed at the skin surface simultaneously in such a way as to target a fraction of the overall surface area while sparing the intervening areas of skin. Confluent epidermal damage is thus avoided. Mechanism of action is via initial induction of proinflammatory cytokines followed by dermal remodeling and collagen induction.[16] Re-epithelialization is observed after as early as 1 day, leading to reduced downtime and higher patient satisfaction.

First fractional lasers were nonablative using midinfrared Erbium-doped fiber lasers. However, the technology base has broadened to include a number of ablative and nonablative fractionated lasers such as 532 nm diode, 850 to 1350 nm infrared, 1064 to 2940 nm Er:YAG, 2790 nm yttrium scandium gallium garnet (YSGG), and 10,600 nm CO_2. The exact technique and device parameters, including microablation spot size and density, are highly variable and are physician- and device-dependent. No ideal fractionation pattern has been established to date. These lasers have demonstrated efficacy in improvement of surgical and traumatic atrophic and hypertrophic scars (see **Figs. 2** and **4**).[17,18] The chief advantage of these lasers is their superior adverse effect profile compared with conventional ablative lasers, including lower risk of scarring and dyspigmentation, along with proven effectiveness.

Timing of Treatment

Most reconstructive surgical interventions are focused on timing with respect to return of tissue

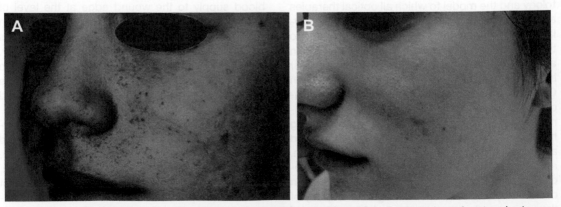

Fig. 2. Patient with scar after angiofibroma excision treated by pulsed dye and Er:YAG laser fractional rejuvenation. (*A*) Before treatment. (*B*) After 1 treatment.

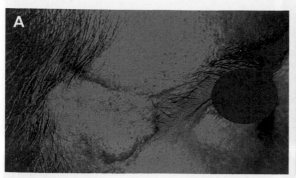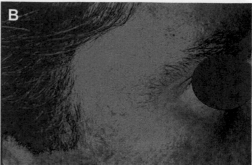

Fig. 3. Hypervascular scar treated using the pulsed dye laser. (*A*) Before treatment. (*B*) After 3 treatments.

mechanical stability. Conventional laser resurfacing and mechanical dermabrasion can potentially destabilize a healing tissue bed or disrupt protective epidermal barrier before the incision seals. Therefore the optimal time for treatment is during the premature phase of scar formation at approximately 6 to 8 weeks after injury. Newer nonablative, pulsed, or fractionated lasers place minimal mechanical stress on the tissues, making an argument for earlier treatments. Earlier intervention can in theory alter the inflammatory phase of wound healing and change fibroblast migration, leading to a reduction in the appearance of scars. Additionally, alterations in microcirculation of the wound induced by laser treatment may be responsible for prevention of excessive scar formation at the incision line.

Benefits of early treatment with PDL for prevention of traumatic and surgical scars were initially demonstrated in a study by McGraw and colleagues[19] in 1999. Treatment within the first few weeks resulted in faster resolution of scar stiffness and erythema, and less frequent development of hypertrophic scarring. Moreover, excellent color blending of the treated scars was obtained after treatment. Other studies have since confirmed the benefits of treatment as early as the time of suture removal.[20,21] Initial consensus recommendations for nonablative fractional laser Fraxel (Reliant Technologies Incorporated, Mountain View, CA, USA) included treatment at 2 to 4 weeks after injury/postoperatively.[22] Results of early treatment with fractional laser are depicted in **Figs. 5** and **6**, with parameters listed in **Table 1**.

Further development of the concept of early interference has led to the development of LASH. This was first proposed by Capon and colleagues[4] in 2001 using an 815 nm diode laser. In animal subjects, they demonstrated accelerated healing with an earlier continuous dermis and epidermis, resulting in a less discernible scar. Tensile strength was significantly greater than control at 7 and 15 days. Clinical trials have affirmed this result, and benefits of the use of this technique in a known hypertrophic scar former have also been demonstrated since the pilot study.[23–25] These preliminary results seem encouraging, but further clinical studies to confirm the effects and to elucidate the exact mechanisms of action are warranted.

Treatment of Traumatic Tattoos

Inadequate primary cleansing of dirt-ingrained skin abrasions can result in disfiguring traumatic tattoos. The resultant discoloration has been successfully treated with excision, dermabrasion, salabrasion, overgrafting, cryotherapy, and microsurgical removal, in addition to optical treatments. Laser treatment of collagen-entrapped pigmented particles takes advantage of selective photothermolysis principle. As such, it is theorized that selective absorption of thermal energy by the entrapped particles leads to shattering of the particles into numerous smaller particles that are subsequently

Table 1 Author parameters for laser devices	
Device	**Parameters**
Pulsed dye laser	Low fluence (4 to 5 J/cm^2), short pulse (0.45 ms), large spot 10 to 12 mm, 30/30 DCD, starting 2 to 4 weeks after suture removal, 4- to 6- week treatment intervals
Sciton Profractional	250–600 μm spot size, 20% to 30% coverage, starting 2 to 4 weeks after suture removal, 4- to 6-week treatment intervals
Fraxel Re:Store	20 mJ and 32% density, starting 2 weeks after suture removal, 4 to 6 treatments at 2-week intervals

Abbreviation: DCD, dynamic cooling device.

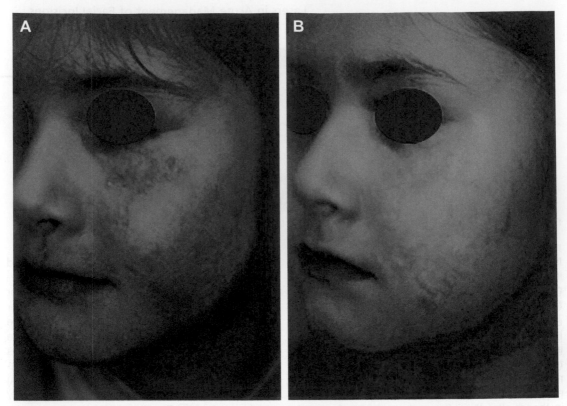

Fig. 4. Dog bite scar treated by Er:YAG Profractional laser. (*A*) Before treatment. (*B*) After 2 treatments.

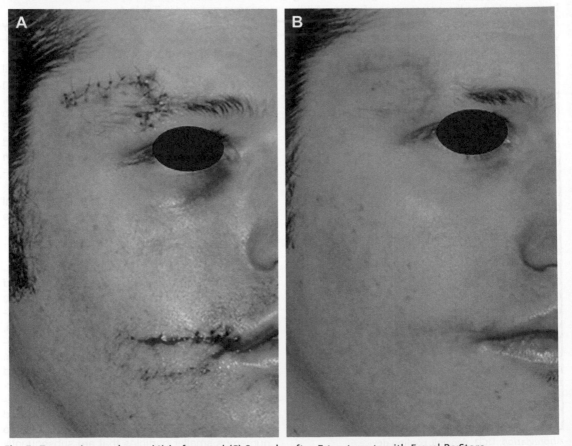

Fig. 5. Traumatic scar shown (*A*) before and (*B*) 2 weeks after 5 treatments with Fraxel Re:Store.

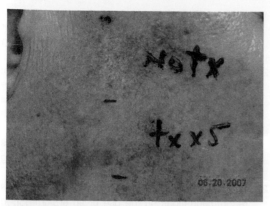

Fig. 6. Another traumatic scar. Lower half of the scar is shown after 5 treatments with Fraxel

phagocytosed and removed by macrophages. Q-switching is a laser technology with widespread use in removal of elective tattoos that allows production of high peak powered pulses with extremely short nanosecond pulse durations. Q-switched ruby, alexandrite, and Nd-YAG lasers have all been demonstrated as effective treatment modalities for traumatic tattoos.[26–29] Repeated treatments, spaced apart by a minimum of 1 month, may be necessary.

Adverse Effects and Complications of Laser Treatment

Despite relative safety and efficacy of laser scar revision, adverse effects and complications may arise that the treating clinician must be aware of and manage. As previously described, conventional CO_2 laser resurfacing can lead to a significant thermal damage to tissues. Continuous wave lasers, in particular the CO_2 lasers, carry the risk of scarring due to considerable collateral thermal damage and necrosis. Hypertrophic scarring is a rare complication of treatment often caused by poor intraoperative technique, and it is treated with topical or intralesional steroids or PDL. Intense postoperative erythema lasting up to 6 months after treatment is an indicator of the degree of nonspecific tissue injury. Intensity and duration are most pronounced with conventional CO_2 lasers. In addition to the erythema, complete epidermal ablation produces an exposed weeping wound along with edema, pain, and pruritis during the initial week after treatment. These symptoms can be managed with cold compresses, pain control, steroids, and antihistamines. Irritation of the skin at this stage can also lead to acne eruptions and contact dermatitis. Infectious complications include reactivation of herpes simplex virus and bacterial and fungal infections. Close monitoring and appropriate antibiotic/antiviral treatment and

preoperative prophylaxis for herpetic infection can minimize the incidence and adverse sequelae of these infections. Postinflammatory hyperpigmentation can complicate recovery of patients with darker skin types and is generally managed with topical bleaching agents, steroids, and retin-A. Incidence of complications can be substantially reduced with careful patient selection, preoperative planning, and meticulous treatment technique. Early detection and treatment of complications is the key to circumventing poor treatment outcomes.

SUMMARY

An unsightly scar negatively affects patients as an unwelcome and often public reminder of a traumatic incident or surgical procedure. Conventional CO_2 is a powerful tool for nonsurgical revision of traumatic and surgical scars, promising excellent results. Unfortunately, the extended recovery period and the adverse effect profile of the treatments make some patients hesitate to undergo this treatment. Newer targeted therapies such as PDL, fractional laser, and nonablative lasers have moderate adverse effect profiles and rapid recovery periods while striving to achieve cosmetic results that approach conventional CO_2 laser resurfacing via earlier interventions.

REFERENCES

1. Katz BE, Oca AG. A controlled study of the effectiveness of spot dermabrasion (scarabrasion) on the appearance of surgical scars. J Am Acad Dermatol 1991;24(3):462 6.
2. Harmon CB, Zelickson BD, Roenigk RK, et al. Dermabrasive scar revision. Immunohistochemical and ultrastructural evaluation. Dermatol Surg 1995;21(6):503–8.
3. Oliveira GV, Hawkins HK, Chinkes D, et al. Hypertrophic versus nonhypertrophic scars compared by immunohistochemistry and laser confocal microscopy: type I and III collagens. Int Wound J 2009;6(6):445–52.
4. Capon A, Souil E, Gauthier B, et al. Laser-assisted skin closure (LASC) by using a 815-nm diode-laser system accelerates and improves wound healing. Lasers Surg Med 2001;28(2):168–75.
5. Cotton J, Hood AF, Gonin R, et al. Histologic evaluation of preauricular and postauricular human skin after high-energy, short-pulse carbon dioxide laser. Arch Dermatol 1996;132(4):425–8.
6. Kitzmiller WJ, Visscher M, Page DA, et al. A controlled evaluation of dermabrasion versus CO_2 laser resurfacing for the treatment of perioral wrinkles. Plast Reconstr Surg 2000;106(6):1366–72 [discussion: 1373–4].

7. Nehal KS, Levine VJ, Ross B, et al. Comparison of high-energy pulsed carbon dioxide laser resurfacing and dermabrasion in the revision of surgical scars. Dermatol Surg 1998;24(6):647–50.

8. Green HA, Domankevitz Y, Nishioka NS. Pulsed carbon dioxide laser ablation of burned skin: in vitro and in vivo analysis. Lasers Surg Med 1990;10(5):476–84.

9. Newman JB, Lord JL, Ash K, et al. Variable pulse erbium:YAG laser skin resurfacing of perioral rhytides and side-by-side comparison with carbon dioxide laser. Lasers Surg Med 2000;26(2):208–14.

10. Anderson RR, Parrish JA. Selective photothermolysis: precise microsurgery by selective absorption of pulsed radiation. Science 1983;220(4596):524–7.

11. Allison KP, Kiernan MN, Waters RA, et al. Pulsed dye laser treatment of burn scars. Alleviation or irritation? Burns 2003;29(3):207–13.

12. Zhibo X, Miaobo Z. Molecular mechanism of pulsed-dye laser in treatment of keloids: an in vitro study. Adv Skin Wound Care 2010;23(1):29–33.

13. Alster TS. Improvement of erythematous and hypertrophic scars by the 585-nm flashlamp-pumped pulsed dye laser. Ann Plast Surg 1994;32(2):186–90.

14. Tong AK, Tan OT, Boll J, et al. Ultrastructure: effects of melanin pigment on target specificity using a pulsed dye laser (577 nm). J Invest Dermatol 1987;88(6):747–52.

15. Manstein D, Herron GS, Sink RK, et al. Fractional photothermolysis: a new concept for cutaneous remodeling using microscopic patterns of thermal injury. Lasers Surg Med 2004;34(5):426–38.

16. Orringer JS, Rittie L, Baker D, et al. Molecular mechanisms of nonablative fractionated laser resurfacing. Br J Dermatol 2010;163(4):757–68.

17. Hunzeker CM, Weiss ET, Geronemus RG. Fractionated CO_2 laser resurfacing: our experience with more than 2000 treatments. Aesthet Surg J 2009;29(4):317–22.

18. Haedersdal M. Fractional ablative CO(2) laser resurfacing improves a thermal burn scar. J Eur Acad Dermatol Venereol 2009;23(11):1340–1.

19. McCraw JB, McCraw JA, McMellin A, et al. Prevention of unfavorable scars using early pulse dye laser treatments: a preliminary report. Ann Plast Surg 1999;42(1):7–14.

20. Conologue TD, Norwood C. Treatment of surgical scars with the cryogen-cooled 595 nm pulsed dye laser starting on the day of suture removal. Dermatol Surg 2006;32(1):13–20.

21. Nouri K, Jimenez GP, Harrison-Balestra C, et al. 585-nm pulsed dye laser in the treatment of surgical scars starting on the suture removal day. Dermatol Surg 2003;29(1):65–73 [discussion: 73].

22. Sherling M, Friedman PM, Adrian R, et al. Consensus recommendations on the use of an erbium-doped 1550-nm fractionated laser and its applications in dermatologic laser surgery. Dermatol Surg 2010;36(4):461–9.

23. Capon A, Iarmarcovai G, Gonnelli D, et al. Scar prevention using laser-assisted skin healing (LASH) in plastic surgery. Aesthetic Plast Surg 2010;34(4):438–46.

24. Capon A, Iarmarcovai G, Mordon S. Laser-assisted skin healing (LASH) in hypertrophic scar revision. J Cosmet Laser Ther 2009;11(4):220–3.

25. Choe JH, Park YL, Kim BJ, et al. Prevention of thyroidectomy scar using a new 1550 nm fractional erbium–glass laser. Dermatol Surg 2009;35(8):1199–205.

26. Achauer BM, Nelson JS, Vander Kam VM, et al. Treatment of traumatic tattoos by Q-switched ruby laser. Plast Reconstr Surg 1994;93(2):318–23.

27. Chang SE, Choi JH, Moon KC, et al. Successful removal of traumatic tattoos in Asian skin with a Q-switched alexandrite laser. Dermatol Surg 1998;24(12):1308–11.

28. Dufresne RG Jr, Garrett AB, Bailin PL, et al. CO_2 laser treatment of traumatic tattoos. J Am Acad Dermatol 1989;20(1):137–8.

29. Haywood RM, Monk BE, Mahaffey PJ. Treatment of traumatic tattoos with the Nd YAG laser: a series of nine cases. Br J Plast Surg 1999;52(2):97–8.

Topical Modalities for Treatment and Prevention of Postsurgical Hypertrophic Scars

Chong Wee Foo, MD*, Payam Tristani-Firouzi, MD

KEYWORDS

- Topical treatment scar • Hypertrophic scar • Vitamin E
- Onion extract • Silicone gel sheets • Imiquimod
- Massage • Pressure garments

Key Points

- There is no single, optimal topical modality that can eliminate or prevent hypertrophic scars.
- Silicone gel sheeting (SGS) remains the most accepted modality in the treatment and prevention of hypertrophic scar.
- Onion extract and vitamin E have not been shown to consistently improve scar appearance as single agents.
- Topical imiquimod 5% cream in a small study was shown to improve scarring.
- Pressure therapy is described predominantly for management of postburn scars.
- Massage therapy is a common modality in the management of scarring in patients with burns, but scientific evidence for its efficacy is limited.

Any cutaneous injury, including surgical incisions, that extends into the dermis will always heal with a scar. The wound healing process is a complex hierarchy of events centered on inflammation, cell proliferation, and remodeling. Cutaneous wounds occasionally heal with scarring that is in excess of what is considered to be a normal physiologic scar. This exuberant scarring results in hypertrophic scars and keloids. Both types of scars are raised, initially pink to purple lesions that are often painful or pruritic. Clinically,

hypertrophic scars are limited to the area of original injury with a tendency toward gradual resolution in time. Keloids extend beyond the original wound margin and seldom resolve spontaneously.

Hypertrophic scars are caused by a variety of factors including mechanical forces on the healing wound (excess tension at wound edge, improper suture placement), poor wound healing, bleeding, or infections. Therapeutic modalities for the prevention and management of scars have been postulated to act by correction of abnormal collagen

---

The authors have no actual or potential conflict of interest, including employment, consultancies, stock ownership, honoraria, patent applications/registrations, grants, or other funding.

Department of Dermatology, University of Utah, 4A330 School of Medicine, 30 North 1900 East, Salt Lake City, UT 84132-2409, USA

* Corresponding author.
E-mail address: chong.foo@hsc.utah.edu

Facial Plast Surg Clin N Am 19 (2011) 551–557
doi:10.1016/j.fsc.2011.06.008
1064-7406/11/$ – see front matter © 2011 Elsevier Inc. All rights reserved.

metabolism, alteration of the immune/inflammatory response, or manipulation of the mechanical properties of wound repair.[1] This article focuses on topical treatments such as SGS and ointment, onion extract, vitamin E, pressure garment therapy, massage therapy, and topical imiquimod 5% cream in the management of hypertrophic scars.

SGS

Silicone polymers are inert, mixed inorganic-organic polymers with a wide array of forms and applications. Polydimethylsiloxane is the most widely used silicon polymer, including in medical products such as SGS. The mechanism of action of SGS is uncertain, but has been postulated to be caused by hydration and occlusion,[2,3] increased oxygen tension,[4,5] and the production of a local static field,[6,7] all of which result in improved remodeling of the scar. The beneficial effects of SGS were first shown in 1983 by Perkins and colleagues[8] in patients with burn scars and contractures. In a controlled study comparing SGS and nonsilicone gel dressing, de Oliveira and colleagues[9] reported improvement in size and induration of hypertrophic scars and keloids in both groups compared with control, but there was no significant difference in results between SGS and nonsilicone gel dressing groups. This finding further suggests that the mechanism of SGS is related to hydration and occlusion.

Several studies have been reported to show clinical efficacy in the treatment of hypertrophic scars with SGS. Ahn and colleagues[10] reported clinical and elastometric improvement of hypertrophic burn scars treated with SGS for 8 weeks compared with untreated scars. The improvement in scar volume lasted up to 6 months. Momeni and colleagues[11] performed a randomized, double-blind, placebo-controlled split-scar trial involving 38 people with hypertrophic burn scars. Using the modified Vancouver Scar Scale, he showed an improvement in pigmentation, vascularity, pliability, and pruritus of treated scars after 4 months of treatment. A prospective controlled study investigating 42 patients with 47 hypertrophic scars comparing 2 types of SGS with no treatment showed improvement in scar color and induration in the treatment group.[12] However, in the study by de Oliveira and colleagues,[9] who compared SGS with nonsilicone gel sheets, there was no difference in scar size or induration between the 2 groups.

The usefulness of SGS in the prevention of scar formation has also been shown. In a prospective study of 20 women with bilateral reduction mammaplasties, patients were instructed to use SGS to 1 breast for 12 hours each day for 2 months.[13] At 2 months, 60% of the nontreated scars were hypertrophic and only 25% of the treated scars were hypertrophic (P<.05). Conversely, in another split-scar study of 155 women who underwent reduction mammaplasties, comparing SGS and nonocclusive Micropore (3M, Ad Leiden, The Netherlands), there were no difference in the occurrence of hypertrophic scarring between the SGS-treated and untreated portions of the scars.[14] Gold and colleagues[15] treated 96 patients who had undergone skin surgery with routine postoperative care or topical SGS for 48 hours after surgery. They showed that patients with a history of abnormal scarring had a lower rate of developing hypertrophic or keloid scar when treated with SGS compared with routine postoperative care (39% vs 71%). In the patients who subsequently underwent scar revision, 36% of patients treated with SGS developed recurrent abnormal scar versus 83% (10 patients) within the routine wound care group. Most recently, in a case series of 7 patients, a liquid silicone gel applied twice a day for 3 months to one-half of a new surgical scar was reported to show noticeable improvement in scar appearance.[16]

In a meta-analysis of SGS for the prevention or treatment of hypertrophic or keloid scars, SGS was found to reduce the incidence of hypertrophic scarring for individuals prone to scarring (relative risk [RR], 0.46; 95% confidence interval [CI], 0.21–0.98).[17] Overall, a significant reduction in scar thickness (RR, −1.99; 95% CI, −2.13 to −1.85) and color amelioration (RR, 3.05; 95% CI, 1.57–5.96) was observed. However, the studies reviewed were deemed highly susceptible to bias. In 2002, an international advisory panel after reviewing more than 300 published articles recommended SGS as a primary option in the management of hypertrophic or keloid scars.[18]

Based on our review of current published studies on SGS, this modality should be considered in the treatment and prevention of hypertrophic scars. The authors typically advise the patients with the earliest signs of hypertrophic scaring to use over-the-counter (OTC) SGS sheets daily for up to 2 months as tolerated. Based on our experience, there are minimal risks, and there is improvement in scar thickness.

VITAMIN E

Vitamin E is a family of essential micronutrients composed of lipid-soluble tocopherols and tocotrienols with strong antioxidant activity. The proposed mechanism of action of vitamin E in modulation of wound healing and scar formation is inhibition of collagen synthesis, and it reduces both fibroblast proliferation and inflammation.[19,20] It is used by the general population to treat wounds, burns, and surgical incisions, with the belief that it improves the cosmetic outcome of scars. In a double-blinded, controlled study, 15 patients who had undergone skin cancer removal surgery applied Aquaphor with and without vitamin E to their wounds twice daily for 4 weeks.[21] In 90% of the cases in this study, topical vitamin E either had no effect on, or worsened, the cosmetic appearance of scars. Of the patients studied, 33% developed a contact dermatitis to the vitamin E. A study of 159 operative procedures for postburn contractures treated postoperatively for 4 months with topical vitamin E showed no beneficial effect in cosmetic appearance or reducing scar formation, but was associated with increased adverse reactions.[22] In a recent prospective, randomized, double-blinded study on 122 patients with surgical scars less than 2 weeks old, topical tocotrienol twice a day for 6 weeks showed no significant difference in treatment and placebo groups using the Patient and Observer Scar Assessment Scale (POSAS), a photographic scar assessment by 2 independent assessors using a visual analogue scale and laser Doppler imaging (LDI).[23]

A limited number of studies have shown a potential beneficial effect with vitamin E. Eight adult patients with hypertrophic scars and keloids were treated with SGS with and without vitamin E.[24] Using a visual analogue scale, a 50% scar improvement was noted in 95% of patients treated with combined vitamin E and SGS compared with 75% of patients treated with SGS alone; the improvement was statistically significant. In another randomized controlled study a combination lotion of silicone and vitamin E showed significant improvement in scar induration, pigmentation, and erythema compared with placebo.[25] Given that the aforementioned 2 studies used a combination of silicone and vitamin E in the active arm, it is unclear whether the silicone or vitamin E component played a larger role in the improvements seen. In a recent study on children with perioperative topical vitamin E on the incision site showed that 96% of patients treated with topical vitamin E reported good cosmetic results compared with 78% of patients treated with emollients.[26]

Based on our review of current published studies on topical vitamin E, and the lack of scientific evidence, we do not recommend the routine use of topical vitamin E for management and prevention of postsurgical scars. In addition, contact allergy is a potential risk with the use of this agent.

ONION EXTRACT

Allium cepa (onion extract) is a common ingredient in several commonly used OTC scar therapy agents. *A cepa* has been found to contain both antibacterial and fibrinolytic activity.[27,28] Mederma (Contractubex, Merz, Frankfurt, Germany), is a topical gel containing 10% aqueous *A cepa* as the active ingredient. The other components of Contractubex gel are 50 IU heparin per gram of gel and 1% allantoin. A few studies have examined the potential effects of onion extract in treatment of surgical scars. In an open trial of Contractubex gel in patients with surgical wounds after thoracic surgery, Willitel and colleagues[29] reported a reduced scar width and reduced frequent of hypertrophic and keloidal scars in the treatment group. In a separate study, Ho and colleagues[30] evaluated the efficacy of Contractubex gel in the prevention of scarring after laser removal of tattoos in 120 Chinese patients. They reported a lower rate of scarring in the treatment group (11.5% in the treatment group vs 23.5% in the control group). Koc and colleagues[31] studied the combination of intralesional triamcinolone and topical onion extract gel versus intralesional triamcinolone alone in 27 patients with keloid or hypertrophic scars of 1 year or more in duration. They reported that intralesional triamcinolone with topical onion extract was more effective than intralesional triamcinolone alone in pain sensitiveness, itching, and elevation but not in erythema and induration. This study was not blinded and lacked a placebo-controlled arm. Campanati and colleagues[32] studied the effect of topical onion extract gel in 30 patients with hypertrophic or keloid scars using intravital videocapillaroscopy, and reported significant reduction in neoangiogenetic features, shown by an improvement in erythema and all videocapillaroscopic markers of neoangiogenesis. In another blinded, placebo-controlled study, 60 postshave excision sites were treated with an onion extract gel. Onion extract treatment resulted in improvements in scar redness, pliability, texture, and the global appearance.[33] Perez and colleagues[25] reported that significant improvements were obtained with onion extract in volume, length, width, and induration of hypertrophic and keloidal scars with a combination of onion extract gel and 0.5% hydrocortisone.

Jackson and colleagues[34] studied 17 patients with surgical scars resulting from Mohs surgery who were treated with topical onion extract or petrolatum-based ointment from suture removal for 1 month. They reported no statistically significant difference between pretreatment and posttreatment evaluations of scar erythema and pruritus in patients using topical onion extract gel. Instead, a statistically significant reduction in scar erythema was found in patients using a petrolatum-based ointment. A subsequent prospective randomized, double-blinded, split-scar study comparing topical onion extract gel and petrolatum-based ointment in 24 patients with new surgical wounds after Mohs or excisional surgery also found no significant difference in scar erythema, hypertrophy, or overall cosmetic appearance.[35]

Review of the published studies on the usefulness of onion extract shows weak to no significant improvement for prevention and improvement in hypertrophic scarring. In addition, many of the reported studies lack a proper control arm. The authors do not routinely recommend the use of these agents in their clinical practice.

IMIQUIMOD 5% CREAM

Topical imiquimod 5% cream is an immunomodulator that is currently approved for the treatment of genital warts, actinic keratosis, and superficial basal cell carcinomas.[36] The mechanism of action is believed to be via induction of interferons resulting in collagen breakdown locally at the site of application and alteration of apoptotic genes.[37] Topical imiquimod has been reported to decrease the recurrence of excised keloids.[38–40] A randomized, double-blinded, placebo-controlled study of imiquimod 5% cream in the prevention of hypertrophic scarring after breast surgery in 15 patients reported improved scar quality compared with control groups (treatment with petrolatum and no treatment).[41] In addition, there was no development of hypertrophic scars or keloids in the patients treated with imiquimod. The main limitation of this

study is the small sample size. Imiquimod treatment of 6 weeks has also been shown to improve the cosmetic outcome of scars after curettage of basal cell carcinomas.[42] Local skin reactions including erythema, edema, ulceration, scaling, and hypopigmentation are common, and can be seen in more than 75% of patients. From 1% to 2% of patient may experience flulike symptoms such as headache, myalgias, fatigue, fever, and diarrhea. These side effects limit the routine use of topical imiquimod in the treatment and prevention of hypertrophic scars. Additional studies are necessary to determine the role of topical imiquimod in scar therapy.

PRESSURE GARMENT THERAPY

Pressure therapy is generally accepted as one of the best nonsurgical means of preventing and controlling hypertrophic scarring after burn injury. The prevalence of hypertrophic scarring after burns was estimated to be about 67% in a single-center retrospective study.[43] The garments are typically custom-made from an elastic material and are intended to be worn for approximately 1 year during the active process of scar maturation.[44] The mechanism of action is uncertain, but is postulated to be related to thinning of the dermis, decrease in edema, and reduction of blood flow resulting in a hypoxic environment with decreased collagen synthesis.[45] The first study to report clinical efficacy of compression pressure garments to treat burn hypertrophic burn scars was in children.[46]

Table 1
Outcomes of topical treatments for scars

Therapy	Potential Pros	Potential Cons	Expert Opinion from this Review
Vitamin E	May improve cosmetic appearance	Contact dermatitis in >30% of patients	Insufficient evidence to recommend
SGS	Prevent hypertrophic scars; scars are flatter and less red	None reported	Recommend
Onion extract	May prevent hypertrophic scars; may improve cosmetic appearance	None reported	Insufficient evidence to recommend
Imiquimod cream	Prevent hypertrophic scars and keloids; may improve cosmetic appearance	Local skin adverse reaction; flulike symptoms	Insufficient evidence to recommend
Pressure garments	May prevent hypertrophic scars after burn injury; scars are flatter and less sensitive	Discomfort from wearing garments for long periods of time	May be used in burn injury; insufficient evidence to recommend for other types of scars
Massage therapy	May reduce pain and itching	None reported	Insufficient evidence to recommend

This was followed by a larger study in Singapore of 280 patients with burns and hypertrophic scars, where pressure garments were shown to result in soft, pliable scars with relief from pain and itch.[47] In a Belgian study, 60 patients with 76 hypertrophic burn scars were assigned to 2 different levels of pressure therapy (mean value of 15 mm Hg vs 10 mm Hg).[48] Scars that were treated with higher pressure garments (15 mm Hg) had a significantly lower scar thickness than scars treated with a lower pressure (10 mm Hg).

A recent meta-analysis was unable to show a difference between global assessments of scars treated with pressure garment therapy and control scars (weighted mean differences, −0.46; 95% CI, −1.07 to 0.16].[39] The meta-analysis for scar height showed a small, but statistically significant, decrease in height for the group treated with pressure garment therapy (standardized mean differences, −0.31; 95% CI, −0.63 to 0.00). Results of meta-analyses of secondary outcome measures of scar vascularity, pliability, and color failed to show a difference between groups. The investigators concluded that the beneficial effects of PGT remain unproven, whereas the discomfort of wearing pressure garments and the cost are significant.

MASSAGE THERAPY

Massage therapy is frequently used in rehabilitation centers in the treatment of burns and scars. Cutaneous hydration, cutaneous mobilization, and pulpar massage are techniques specifically cited to manage hypertrophic scars and keloids. Although massage therapy has been reported to improve pain, itching, and anxiety,[49,50] there have been few studies of its clinical efficacy in treating scars. In a study of 30 children with hypertrophic burn scars, frictional massage combined with pressure garments were compared with pressure garments alone.[51] The study failed to show any appreciable effects of massage therapy on the vascularity, pliability, and height of the hypertrophic scars studied. Because of the limited number of studies available on this subject; we are unable to make any recommendations on the use of massage therapy in the treatment of scars. However, the authors routinely recommend massaging to prevent the risk of postsurgical hypertrophic scars. Patients are instructed to start massaging 4 weeks after surgery, 2 to 3 times daily for 3 to 5 minutes after application of either petrolatum or moisturizing cream for 3 to 4 months. In their experience, this simple regimen results in improvement in scar thickness and contour.

SUMMARY

There is no universally accepted treatment regimen and no evidence-based literature to guide the management of hypertrophic scars. Leventhal and colleagues[52] reviewed 70 treatment modalities in a meta-analysis and estimated the overall success rate to be approximately 60%, with no statistically significant difference between different therapies. In conclusion, there is no single, optimal topical modality that can eliminate or prevent hypertrophic scars. SGS remains the most accepted modality for the treatment and prevention of hypertrophic scar. There are minimal data to support the direct benefit of onion extract and vitamin E as single agents. Pressure therapy and massage therapy are predominately used for treatment of burn scars. Topical imiquimod 5% cream in a small study was shown to improve scarring and requires further clinical studies. **Table 1** gives a summary of the agents and the authors' experience with outcomes.

REFERENCES

1. Cohen IK, McCoy BJ. The biology and control of surface overhealing. World J Surg 1980;4(3): 289–95.
2. Sawada Y, Sone K. Hydration and occlusion treatment for hypertrophic scars and keloids. Br J Plast Surg 1992;45(8):599–603.
3. Chang CC, Kuo YF, Chiu HC, et al. Hydration, not silicone, modulates the effects of keratinocytes on fibroblasts. J Surg Res 1995;59(6):705–11.
4. Gilman TH. Silicone sheet for treatment and prevention of hypertrophic scar: a new proposal for the mechanism of efficacy. Wound Repair Regen 2003; 11(3):235–6.
5. Brown NJ, Smyth EA, Cross SS, et al. Angiogenesis induction and regression in human surgical wounds. Wound Repair Regen 2002;10(4):245–51.
6. Hirshowitz B, Lindenbaum E, Har-Shai Y, et al. Static-electric field induction by a silicone cushion for the treatment of hypertrophic and keloid scars. Plast Reconstr Surg 1998;101(5):1173–83.
7. Amicucci G, Schietroma M, Rossi M, et al. Silicone occlusive sheeting vs silicone cushion for the treatment of hypertrophic and keloid scars. A prospective-randomized study. Ann Ital Chir 2005;76(1):79–83 [in Italian].
8. Perkins K, Davey RB, Wallis KA. Silicone gel: a new treatment for burn scars and contractures. Burns Incl Therm Inj 1983;9(3):201–4.
9. de Oliveira GV, Nunes TA, Magna LA, et al. Silicone versus nonsilicone gel dressings: a controlled trial. Dermatol Surg 2001;27(8):721–6.

10. Ahn ST, Monafo WW, Mustoe TA. Topical silicone gel: a new treatment for hypertrophic scars. Surgery 1989;106(4):781–6 [discussion: 6–7].

11. Momeni M, Hafezi F, Rahbar H, et al. Effects of silicone gel on burn scars. Burns 2009;35(1): 70–4.

12. Carney SA, Cason CG, Gowar JP, et al. Cica-Care gel sheeting in the management of hypertrophic scarring. Burns 1994;20(2):163–7.

13. Cruz-Korchin NI. Effectiveness of silicone sheets in the prevention of hypertrophic breast scars. Ann Plast Surg 1996;37(4):345–8.

14. Niessen FB, Spauwen PH, Robinson PH, et al. The use of silicone occlusive sheeting (Sil-K) and silicone occlusive gel (Epiderm) in the prevention of hypertrophic scar formation. Plast Reconstr Surg 1998;102(6):1962–72.

15. Gold MH, Foster TD, Adair MA, et al. Prevention of hypertrophic scars and keloids by the prophylactic use of topical silicone gel sheets following a surgical procedure in an office setting. Dermatol Surg 2001; 27(7):641–4.

16. Spencer JM. Case series: evaluation of a liquid silicone gel on scar appearance following excisional surgery–a pilot study. J Drugs Dermatol 2010;9(7): 856–8.

17. O'Brien L, Pandit A. Silicon gel sheeting for preventing and treating hypertrophic and keloid scars. Cochrane Database Syst Rev 2006;(1):CD003826.

18. Mustoe TA, Cooter RD, Gold MH, et al. International clinical recommendations on scar management. Plast Reconstr Surg 2002;110(2):560–71.

19. Ehrlich HP, Tarver H, Hunt TK. Inhibitory effects of vitamin E on collagen synthesis and wound repair. Ann Surg 1972;175(2):235–40.

20. Musalmah M, Fairuz AH, Gapor MT, et al. Effect of vitamin E on plasma malondialdehyde, antioxidant enzyme levels and the rates of wound closures during wound healing in normal and diabetic rats. Asia Pac J Clin Nutr 2002;11(Suppl 7):S448–51.

21. Baumann LS, Spencer J. The effects of topical vitamin E on the cosmetic appearance of scars. Dermatol Surg 1999;25(4):311–5.

22. Jenkins M, Alexander JW, MacMillan BG, et al. Failure of topical steroids and vitamin E to reduce postoperative scar formation following reconstructive surgery. J Burn Care Rehabil 1986;7(4):309–12.

23. Khoo TL, Halim AS, Zakaria Z, et al. A prospective, randomised, double-blinded trial to study the efficacy of topical tocotrienol in the prevention of hypertrophic scars. J Plast Reconstr Aesthet Surg 2011; 64(6):e137–45.

24. Palmieri B, Gozzi G, Palmieri G. Vitamin E added silicone gel sheets for treatment of hypertrophic scars and keloids. Int J Dermatol 1995;34(7):506–9.

25. Perez OA, Viera MH, Patel JK, et al. A comparative study evaluating the tolerability and efficacy of two

topical therapies for the treatment of keloids and hypertrophic scars. J Drugs Dermatol 2010;9(5): 514–8.

26. Zampieri N, Zuin V, Burro R. A prospective study in children: pre- and post-surgery use of vitamin E in surgical incisions. J Plast Reconstr Aesthet Surg 2009;63(9):1474–8.

27. Augusti KT. Therapeutic values of onion (Allium cepa L) and garlic (Allium sativum L). Indian J Exp Biol 1996;34(7):634–40.

28. Dankert J, Tromp TF, de Vries H, et al. Antimicrobial activity of crude juices of Allium ascalonicum, Allium cepa and Allium sativum. Zentralbl Bakteriol Orig A 1979;245(1–2):229–39.

29. Willital GH, Heine H. Efficacy of Contractubex gel in the treatment of fresh scars after thoracic surgery in children and adolescents. Int J Clin Pharmacol Res 1994;14(5–6):193–202.

30. Ho WS, Ying SY, Chan PC, et al. Use of onion extract, heparin, allantoin gel in prevention of scarring in Chinese patients having laser removal of tattoos: a prospective randomized controlled trial. Dermatol Surg 2006;32(7):891–6.

31. Koc E, Arca E, Surucu B, et al. An open, randomized, controlled, comparative study of the combined effect of intralesional triamcinolone acetonide and onion extract gel and intralesional triamcinolone acetonide alone in the treatment of hypertrophic scars and keloids. Dermatol Surg 2008;34(11): 1507–14.

32. Campanati A, Savelli A, Sandroni L, et al. Effect of Allium cepa-allantoin-pentaglycan gel on skin hypertrophic scars: clinical and video-capillaroscopic results of an open-label, controlled, nonrandomized clinical trial. Dermatol Surg 2010;36(9):1439–44.

33. Draelos ZD. The ability of onion extract gel to improve the cosmetic appearance of postsurgical scars. J Cosmet Dermatol 2008;7(2):101–4.

34. Jackson BA, Shelton AJ. Pilot study evaluating topical onion extract as treatment for postsurgical scars. Dermatol Surg 1999;25(4):267–9.

35. Chung VQ, Kelley L, Marra D, et al. Onion extract gel versus petrolatum emollient on new surgical scars: prospective double-blinded study. Dermatol Surg 2006;32(2):193–7.

36. Berman B. Imiquimod: a new immune response modifier for the treatment of external genital warts and other diseases in dermatology. Int J Dermatol 2002;41(Suppl 1):7–11.

37. Jacob SE, Berman B, Nassiri M, et al. Topical application of imiquimod 5% cream to keloids alters expression genes associated with apoptosis. Br J Dermatol 2003;149(Suppl 66):62–5.

38. Berman B, Kaufman J. Pilot study of the effect of postoperative imiquimod 5% cream on the recurrence rate of excised keloids. J Am Acad Dermatol 2002;47(Suppl 4):S209–11.

39. Anzarut A, Olson J, Singh P, et al. The effectiveness of pressure garment therapy for the prevention of abnormal scarring after burn injury: a meta-analysis. J Plast Reconstr Aesthet Surg 2009;62(1):77–84.

40. Malhotra AK, Gupta S, Khaitan BK, et al. Imiquimod 5% cream for the prevention of recurrence after excision of presternal keloids. Dermatology 2007; 215(1):63–5.

41. Prado A, Andrades P, Benitez S, et al. Scar management after breast surgery: preliminary results of a prospective, randomized, and double-blind clinical study with Aldara cream 5% (imiquimod). Plast Reconstr Surg 2005;115(3):966–72.

42. Rigel DS, Torres AM, Ely H. Imiquimod 5% cream following curettage without electrodesiccation for basal cell carcinoma: preliminary report. J Drugs Dermatol 2008;7(1 Suppl 1):s15–6.

43. Bombaro KM, Engrav LH, Carrougher GJ, et al. What is the prevalence of hypertrophic scarring following burns? Burns 2003;29(4):299–302.

44. Puzey G. The use of pressure garments on hypertrophic scars. J Tissue Viability 2002;12(1):11–5.

45. Staley MJ, Richard RL. Use of pressure to treat hypertrophic burn scars. Adv Wound Care 1997; 10(3):44–6.

46. Garcia-Velasco M, Ley R, Mutch D, et al. Compression treatment of hypertrophic scars in burned children. Can J Surg 1978;21(5):450–2.

47. Ng CL, Lee ST, Wong KL. Pressure garments in the prevention and treatment of keloids. Ann Acad Med Singapore 1983;12(Suppl 2):430–5.

48. Van den Kerckhove E, Stappaerts K, Fieuws S, et al. The assessment of erythema and thickness on burn related scars during pressure garment therapy as a preventive measure for hypertrophic scarring. Burns 2005;31(6):696–702.

49. Field T, Peck M, Hernandez-Reif M, et al. Postburn itching, pain, and psychological symptoms are reduced with massage therapy. J Burn Care Rehabil 2000;21(3):189–93.

50. Field T, Peck M, Krugman S, et al. Burn injuries benefit from massage therapy. J Burn Care Rehabil 1998;19(3):241–4.

51. Patino O, Novick C, Merlo A, et al. Massage in hypertrophic scars. J Burn Care Rehabil 1999; 20(3):268–71 [discussion: 267].

52. Leventhal D, Furr M, Reiter D. Treatment of keloids and hypertrophic scars: a meta-analysis and review of the literature. Arch Facial Plast Surg 2006;8(6): 362–8.

Use of Hair Grafting in Scar Camouflage

Lucy Barr, MD[a],*, Alfonso Barrera, MD[b]

KEYWORDS

- Scar camouflage • Hair transplant • Follicular unit grafting
- Hair grafting • Facial scars • Madarosis
- Cicatricial alopecia

Loss of hair-bearing tissue in the head and neck area can result from surgery, trauma, burns, tumors, and infection, as well as a diversity of inflammatory conditions such as lichen plano pilaris, which causes irreversible damage to the hair follicle. The resulting defect can be cosmetically disfiguring and can present a challenging problem for the reconstructive surgeon. Several well-established treatment modalities have been used for reconstruction of these areas including secondary intention, primary closure, local flaps, skin grafts, allografts, free flaps, and hair transplantation.

Hair transplantation can be used as a reconstructive method alone or in conjunction with the other techniques. The use of hair grafts for scar camouflage was used as early as the 1970s,[1] during which punch grafting was the method of treatment. Standard punch grafting is what generally created a "doll's hair" appearance. Hair transplantation has evolved over the decades, and the current method of using follicular unit grafts has led to very natural restorations for a variety of areas including not only the scalp but also the eyebrows, eyelashes, and the beard areas. The hair used for facial hair transplants can be harvested from the occipital and temporal areas, the same donor region as is used for restoration of the scalp.

Norman Orentreich described a key concept called "donor dominance," which has helped to form the foundation of hair restoration. He stated that donor hair characteristics such as texture, color, growth rate, and anagen (growth) period are maintained after transplantation and that the transplanted hair behaves independently of the recipient site. Although the concept of donor dominance is not as straightforward as originally thought, transplanted facial hair will grow with similar properties to that of the donor site, thus requiring trimming and grooming. The camouflage provided by hair grafts can provide a restoration not obtainable with other methods. One's surgical armamentarium will be greatly complemented by offering this technique, affording a more comprehensive approach to treating these patients.

FOLLICULAR UNIT TRANSPLANTATION

Understanding the basic concepts of follicular transplantation is critical when approaching patients requiring reconstruction of scarring in the hair-bearing regions of the head and neck. The concept of the follicular unit was described in 1984[2] and has revolutionized the preparation of the grafts, allowing surgeons to create a much more natural-appearing recipient bed. While studying the horizontal histology of the scalp, it was found that hairs grow in natural groupings of 1, 2, 3, or 4 terminal hairs with their own neurovascular bundles, a piloerectile muscle, sebaceous gland, sweat gland, and subcutaneous fat, all surrounded by a sheath of collagen.[3] Today, as surgeons dissect these follicular units under magnification the aim is to keep them as intact as possible.

The authors have no financial disclosures.
a Barr Facial Plastic Surgery, 24 South 1100 East, Suite 301, Salt Lake City, UT 84121, USA
b Baylor College of Medicine, Plastic and Cosmetic Surgery, 915 Gessner Drive, Suite # 825, Houston, TX 77024-2527, USA
* Corresponding author.
E-mail address: lucyjbarr@gmail.com

Facial Plast Surg Clin N Am 19 (2011) 559–568
doi:10.1016/j.fsc.2011.06.010

Hair transplantation involves aesthetically redistributing follicular units from the donor site to a much larger recipient site with the goal of maximizing the cosmetic impact of the surgery. It is important to recognize that recreating 50% of the native density on the scalp will create an excellent optical cosmetic density. If the demand outweighs the supply, grafts may be "weighted" to improve optical density in more cosmetically important areas such as the front or the side that the hair is combed from. Recipient site density may vary from 20 follicular units/cm^2 to 65 follicular units/cm^2. One needs to balance the desire to create an ideal cosmetic density with the donor supply available as well as the survival of the grafts. It is critical that the patient also understands this concept.

Placing more than 30 follicular units/cm^2 into normal tissue is considered "dense packing"[4] (although this term is variably defined by hair transplant surgeons). Dense packing may risk poor growth of the grafts and even skin necrosis depending on the vascularity of the recipient site. There is some debate regarding what the ideal cosmetic density is, but most would not argue with the safety and cosmetic outcome of creating a density of approximately 35 follicular units/cm^2. In a normally vascularized area the graft survival rate ranges between 90% and 95%. In reconstructive cases, the vascular supply that will support the newly transplanted grafts must be considered. If significantly compromised, one should not dense pack, and the patient and his or her family must be informed that 2 to 3 or even 4 sessions may be necessary for a more optimal result.

To optimally camouflage a scar in the hair-bearing scalp, it is important to understand and recreate patterns found in nature. For a male, the anterior hair line should originate where the vertical forehead changes to horizontal caudal scalp (**Fig. 1**) approximately 8 cm above the glabella.[5] Typically, a slightly flared line then joins the temporal hump laterally at the vertical level of the lateral canthus to create the frontal hairline contour (**Fig. 2**). The design of the female hairline differs from that of the male in that the hairline should start at a height of approximately 5.5 cm above the glabella and frequently has a "widow's peak" and lateral mounds.[6] Hairline design is a topic of continual debate and discussion. Transition zones of 1-hair and 2-hair grafts are used at the hairline with 3-hair and 4-hair grafts preserved for the center of the parietal scalp. Macroirregularity and microirregularity of the grafts are also used in these transition zones to create a natural appearance.[7] When reconstructing a scarred region in the crown, it is important to recognize the whorl patterns that occur naturally. The S-shaped

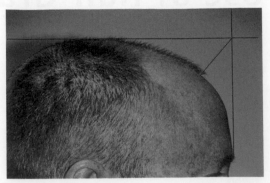

Fig. 1. The male anterior hairline should originate approximately 8 cm above the glabella where the vertical forehead meets the horizontal caudal scalp.

pattern (**Fig. 3**) is the most common pattern seen in Caucasian men.[8] Designing the recipient site is the art of hair restoration. It is critical to pay close attention to the native hair as well as the patient's preferences and styling patterns when creating the design for maximum camouflage.

When developing a treatment plan, one should always consider the patient's personal and family history of androgenic alopecia. A history of advanced balding on either side of the family is a great risk factor for progressive hair loss in the patient as well. When appropriate, scalp recipient sites should always be designed with future hair loss in mind to avoid the cosmetic deformity that can occur as miniaturized hair recedes away

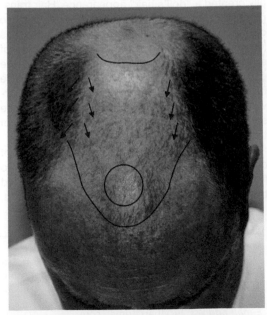

Fig. 2. The frontal hairline meets the temporal hump laterally at the level of the lateral canthus.

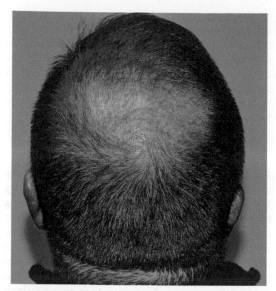

Fig. 3. Hair transplanted into the crown area should mimic what is seen in nature. The S-shape seen in this patient is the most common whorl pattern seen in Caucasian men.

from genetically stable transplanted hair. These patients should be encouraged to start on medical therapy to preserve the hair that they have and, if future hair loss is anticipated, they should be educated about the potential need for more hair grafting as their hair recedes.

Once the recipient site is designed, donor hair is harvested from the occipital scalp in the region just above the external occipital protuberance where the hair is genetically stable (**Fig. 4**). It is in this region where the density is greatest on the scalp is most resistant to hormone-related alopecia. When evaluating the donor site, the length of the donor region can be measured from 3 cm behind the hairline at the temple to a corresponding spot

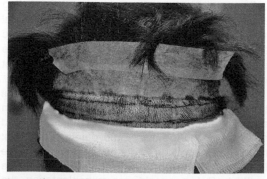

Fig. 4. The donor site is located at the occipital scalp just above the external occipital protuberance where the hair is genetically stable.

on the contralateral side.[9] The hair transplantation surgeon should always keep in mind the limited donor reservoir of good genetic hair available, which is approximately 30 × 4 cm. As a general rule of thumb, half of the donor area may be moved (in total) without a significant change in appearance. Strips measuring less than 1.5 cm in width are less likely to result in a widened scar. The amount of donor hair available is dependent on the density of hair present as well as the laxity of the scalp in the occipital area. These two factors can be compromised by injury and previous scalp surgery. If the scalp has been stretched from previous surgery, the follicular units will be spaced further apart. Scarring in the donor area will also have a significant impact on the ultimate donor yield. It is important to measure the patient's scalp laxity and density to determine the width of the strip that can be harvested to meet the needs of the recipient site.

The harvesting of donor hairs can be performed using either the strip technique or follicular unit extraction.[10] With the strip technique, an appropriately sized elongated ellipse of donor scalp is harvested just deep to the follicles and closed. With follicular unit extraction (FUE), follicular units are directly extracted from the donor area using a small punch that may leave an inconspicuous scar; this may be a better technique for patients who like to wear their hair very short. When donor hair reserves are scarce, FUE may also be used to harvest body hair for grafting, termed body hair transplant.[11] One region where the use of FUE can be helpful is in the case of a wide occipital donor scar. While generally one can prevent a widened donor scar by harvesting long narrow strips, widened scars are still seen, especially in the patient who has undergone multiple hair transplant surgeries in the past. Because of the limited scalp laxity and often depleted donor reserve, FUE is an excellent method for restoration of this scar. Although FUE is an exciting alternative to the strip technique, hair transection on extraction as well as other technical problems exist and thus limit its use by many hair surgeons.

Once the donor hair is harvested, the excess tissue between each unit is dissected away while the germinative and vital support components of each unit are preserved. Hair grafts are free tissue grafts that survive only by anaerobic metabolism. Any desiccation, trauma, or increase in metabolic or ischemia time will influence the final survival rate of the transplanted follicles.[12] Efforts to reduce ischemia-reperfusion injury and improve graft survival have led to experimentation with different storage solutions for the purpose of delayed transplantation. Grafts may be stored in a Petri dish containing 4% saline or lactated Ringer solution; however, there are now other commercially available solutions such as HypoThermosol (BioLife Solutions Inc, Bothell, WA) that contain antioxidants such as vitamin E and glutathione, which may alleviate ischemia-reperfusion injury.[13] Following creation of the follicular units, recipient incisions are made according to the design developed preoperatively, and the hair is transplanted to the recipient area. After the grafts are placed, nutrients from the recipient bed enable survival until circulation is established days later.

As previously mentioned, the concept of donor dominance has formed the foundation of hair restoration; however, it is now understood that the recipient site has some influence on the growth characteristics of transplanted hairs. The cell cycle such as the anagen phase may be influenced by the recipient bed on the background of innate programming of the follicle when hairs are transplanted to sites away from the scalp.[14] This concept becomes more relevant as one continues to graft hair-bearing regions outside of the scalp (ie, the face) with scalp hair.

The face is the second most common area for hair transplantation, and can include eyebrows, eyelashes, moustaches, and beards. It is important to pay attention to the hair patterns present in the recipient site so as to mimic these properties when transplanting hairs to scars in these regions. The hair on the face does not grow in follicular units, and single-hair grafts should be used when transplanting the beard.[15] Two to 3 hair grafts may be used toward the center of the moustache to improve density.

The eyebrows and eyelashes are especially sensitive to the direction of the recipient incision and exit angle of the hair shaft and, hence, growth direction of the hair. The transplanted hair shaft should be left longer to facilitate better control of hair direction during implantation into the recipient site. Donor hair may be taken from the occipital scalp, temple, or other areas such as the postauricular region, brow, and nasal vibrissae, to closer mimic the hair qualities such as shaft diameter and anagen phase duration. In the eyebrow, incisions should be nearly parallel to the skin surface so that the hairs grow almost flat against the skin surface as in natural eyebrows. Mostly 1-hair grafts should be used, although some 2-hair grafts can be placed centrally. When restoring an eyebrow, 150 to 200 grafts may be used per brow with the superiormost hairs angled inferiorly and the inferior edge angled superiorly.[15] For eyelid hair grafts, many techniques are being developed and used by hair restoration surgeons around the world. Depending on technique, approximately

60 hairs per lid may be grafted. The majority of the epithelium should be trimmed off to avoid hordoleum (stye). The incisions may be made in a variety of ways to produce an exit site at the ciliary margin overlapping the original eyelash at an angle of about 30° with the curl of the hair facing upward.[16] Grooming, trimming, and curling of the hairs is typically necessary.

HAIR GRAFTING FOR SCARS

Preventing visible scars in hair-bearing regions is always preferable to requiring a second surgery for scar camouflage. Although good results can be obtained with trichophytic closures, growth of hair through the scar can result in ingrown hairs and irregularity of growth direction. When making incisions parallel to the hair follicles, despite tension-free closures, incisions often leave a visible hairless linear scar. A method that may be used adjunctively is to place hair grafts dissected from the corners of skin after excising a benign lesion that would have otherwise been discarded, and placing them into the newly closed wound to conceal an anticipated scar after a tension-free closure. Once the wound has been closed, hair grafts are dissected using a standard technique from the excised hair-bearing skin; these can then be inserted into the wound in between adjacent sutures using jeweler's forceps. It is not well understood how this may affect the tensile strength of the wound, and it is recommended that sutures be left in place several days longer than usual.[17] This delay saves the patient from a second operation.

Hair grafting for scar camouflage is a critical component of a multimodality approach to scar improvement, and is an accepted part of the standard of care in the reconstruction of scars in hair-bearing areas. Hair grafting can be used alone or in conjunction with other methods such as serial excision or scalp expansion/reduction. Follicular unit transplants have the advantage of creating a hair density and growth direction that is natural in appearance, providing for a more aesthetic and manageable restoration. Overall, the same principles apply as when approaching a patient with androgenic alopecia.

More continues to be learned about optimal techniques as well as their potential application and limitations. Grafting into scar tissue and grafted skin does have some unique obstacles: the blood supply is reduced relative to native tissue, the tissue is stiff, and the skin may not be as thick. Before considering transplantation, the scar tissue should be mature, ideally with some substance and pliability. In addition, hypertrophic or keloid scars should be treated to provide a tissue bed that is at the same level as the surrounding skin prior to transplantation.

When approaching vascularly impaired skin, it is best to err on the cautious side when creating a surgical plan, due to the concern that grafting into a scarred recipient bed may produce a lower survival rate of donor hair. Several investigators have found that because of their small size and low metabolic requirements, hair grafts grow well in scars even in very large areas of burns and thin skin[18–21]; however, care should be taken to minimize further compromising blood supply. Special techniques include limiting the use of epinephrine in the recipient bed as well as leaving the grafts "chubby," with ample subcutaneous tissue surrounding the germinative center of the hair follicle. When grafting into very thin skin and skin grafts, placement of the grafts will need to be at an acute angle in the general direction of natural hair growth, as the tissue bed is very shallow. The use of tumescence and/or fat grafting before the placement of grafts has been used by some surgeons who have anecdotally noted that these techniques may assist in proper placement and optimal growth of grafts in this attenuated tissue. In has been shown that fat grafting improves the clinical appearance of burn scars, with new collagen deposition as well as an increase in vascularity seen on histologic examination.[22] This finding may support the clinical observation of improved hair growth in scar tissue that has previously been fat grafted. Barrera (personal observation) has also noted an improved clinical appearance of the scar, including texture, thickness, and pliability, after transplanting hair grafts directly into scar tissue, an improvement that may be a result of stem cells present in the follicular units. The contribution of stem cells to the field of hair restoration is an active area of research.

Other well-described methods may improve the vascularity of the recipient bed. If the defect location allows, the transposition of a temporalis fascia flap to the site of a thin skin graft will increase the vascularity of the recipient bed, likely improving graft survival of the subsequent hair transplant surgery.[23] Follicular unit grafting has also been used to help camouflage free-flap reconstructions in the lower face of a male. Survival of follicular unit grafts transplanted into free flaps approximates the rate achievable in native scalp.[24]

It was previously discussed that in normal scalp, dense packing can compromise blood supply to the grafts. This aspect should be strongly considered when approaching a scarred tissue bed. Grafts placed using a density of 20 to 30 grafts per cm^2 is reasonable. The use of a higher density

for small scars and a lower density for larger scars is recommended. When grafting at lower densities, a second or third stage will likely be required to obtain ideal cosmetic density. Some surgeons (presentation by Dr Robert Jones at ISHRS meeting, October 2010) will use higher densities when approaching even larger cases, but recommend testing a small area to assess graft survival before proceeding with the entire restoration. When approaching extensive areas of alopecia, it may be wise to consider staging the reconstruction by grafting the most peripheral areas with the best blood supply first and grafting the centermost regions at a second stage. One to 3 sessions over the course of 6 to 18 months will be required to achieve optimal aesthetic results. Alternative techniques including scalp expansion should also be considered in these cases.

CASES AND TECHNIQUE

The use of hair grafting for scar camouflage has a wide variety of applications in the head and neck region, including the hair-bearing regions of the face. Anyone who practices facial plastic surgery is eventually going to see patients who have previously had a browlift or facelift resulting in a distorted hairline with visible scarring. While preventing these scars is more optimal than treating them after they have occurred, the use of hair grafting is an excellent method of restoring these secondary deformities.[25,26] The loss of sideburn and postauricular hair are stigmata of facelift surgeries that interfere with a woman's ability to style her hair freely, and can be aesthetically disturbing to these patients.

In restoring this area, a horizontal ellipse of scalp is harvested from the occipital region. In this case (**Fig. 5**) intravenous sedation was used. The donor site was injected with 0.5% Marcaine with 1:200,000 epinephrine. Tumescent (120 mL normal saline, 20 mL 2% Xilocaine, and 1 mL 1:1000 epinephrine) infiltration is also used prior to strip harvesting to aid in excision. The size of the strip harvested in this case measured 8 × 1 cm and the donor site was closed using a running continuous 3-0 Prolene suture. Under magnification, the grafts were then dissected into individual 1- to 2-hair follicular unit grafts. Incisions to the recipient site were made using a 22.5° Sharpoint blade, which was attached to a Beaver blade handle. This blade has a 22.5° angle of the point of the blade. Care was taken to angle the incisions acutely, consistent with the exit angle of the surrounding hair. A total of 809 grafts were transplanted bilaterally to the sideburn and retroauricular areas using jeweler's forceps to insert the grafts. Single-hair

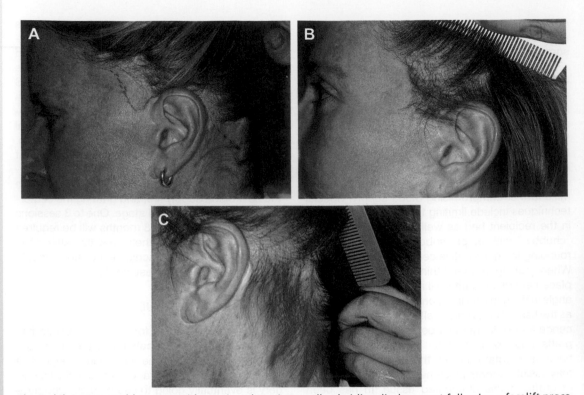

Fig. 5. (*A*) A 55-year-old woman with scarring alopecia as well as hairline displacement following a facelift procedure. (*B, C*) Five months after follicular unit grafting to sideburn and retroauricular area.

grafts were used along the hairline and 2-hair grafts were placed more posteriorly. It is clear from **Fig. 5**C that at 5 months, the patient is starting to have growth of the transplanted hair with a natural-appearing restoration in one surgical stage.

Scarring can occur following repair of the upper lip and philtrum despite optimal surgical technique, such as in repair of the congenital cleft lip. Philtral scars may persist as a region that appears hypopigmented, depressed, and or non–hair bearing.[11,27] The demonstrated case (**Fig. 6**) shows successful grafting to the moustache is this 43-year-old man who underwent bilateral cleft lip repair as well as an Abbe flap. He had a small area of alopecia and a depressed scar. A 3 × 1-cm sized ellipse was harvested from the occipital scalp and closed using 3-0 Prolene. The strip was dissected into 1-hair and 2-hair follicular unit grafts. Recipient incisions were made using a 15° Sharpoint blade, which makes a smaller incision site than the 22.5° blade. Care was taken to avoid injury to the surrounding hair follicles when making the new incisions. Single-hair grafts were used along the superior border of the moustache to provide for additional camouflage. Two-hair grafts were used centrally and through the scar with single-hair grafts at the white roll. In this region, there is less bleeding and less

"popping out" of the grafts if the incisions are made first and grafts placed minutes later. A total of 143 hair grafts were used. Note that the color of the grafted hair is slightly darker than some of the native hair, consistent with the donor dominance theory.

Scarring may also occur in this area from a variety of other causes, as in the patient (**Fig. 7**) who suffered a third-degree burn to the face. This male patient is an excellent candidate for scar camouflage using hair grafting. In this region, 2-hair grafts were used in the center of the mustache with single-hair grafts peripherally. In the chin/beard area, single-hair grafts were used and were placed at a less acute angle, mimicking that of the natural hair on the contralateral side. A total of 407 follicular unit grafts were transplanted in the first session. A second session was performed 12 months later with an additional 430 grafts, for a total of 837 grafts after both procedures.

The patient in **Fig. 7** also suffered a third-degree burn to the left brow area (**Fig. 8**), resulting in cicatricial alopecia of this region. During the same procedure, hairs were used from the same strip to restore the brow. Incisions were made using a 15° Sharpoint blade. A total of 70 grafts were placed using 2-hair grafts centrally and single-hair

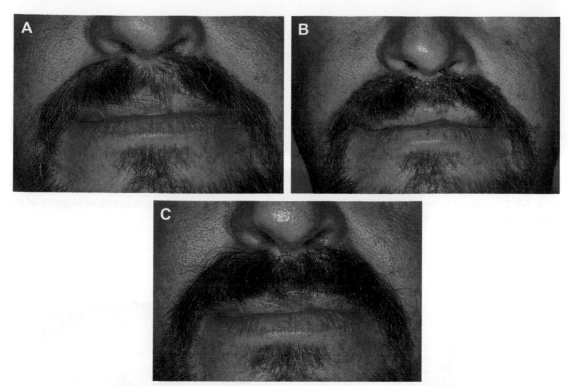

Fig. 6. (*A*) A 43-year-old man, who underwent repair of a cleft lip along with an Abbe flap. He has alopecia in the region of repair. (*B*) Immediately postoperatively with grafts in place. (*C*) One year after 143 follicular unit grafts to the scar and surrounding areas.

grafts on the peripheral aspect of the newly restored brow.

Madarosis can result from trauma or oncologic resection. Hair grafting to the eyelid region requires special instrumentation for stabilizing the lid, creating the recipient sites, and placing the hair grafts. A few different techniques have been described for the placement of follicular units. For this case (**Fig. 9**), a 22.5° Sharpoint blade was used to make the incisions. When performing madarosis cases today, it is preferable to use a smaller incision blade or needle such as a 15° Sharpoint blade or 23F curved needle. These methods create a smaller incision, adequate for 1-hair and 2-hair grafts, and avoid the potential visibility of the incision scar. However, this patient had an acceptable result using the 22.5° blade. A chalazion clamp was used to stabilize the lid margin and protect the globe (see **Fig. 9B**). Thirty-two follicular unit grafts were placed using

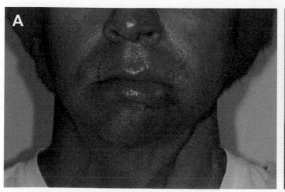
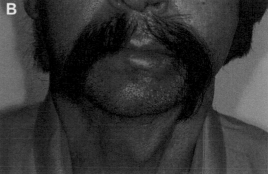

Fig. 7. (*A*) A 42-year-old man who suffered a third-degree burn to the face including the left philtrum and chin. (*B*) One year following 2 stages of follicular unit grafting to the left philtrum and chin. A total of 837 grafts were used.

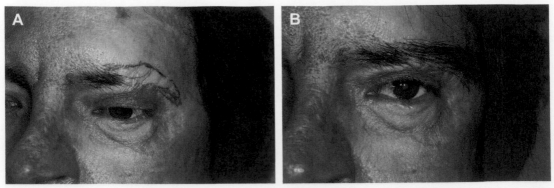

Fig. 8. (*A*) The patient from **Fig. 7** also suffered burn injury to the left brow, resulting in cicatricial alopecia of this region. (*B*) One year after follicular unit reconstruction of left eyebrow.

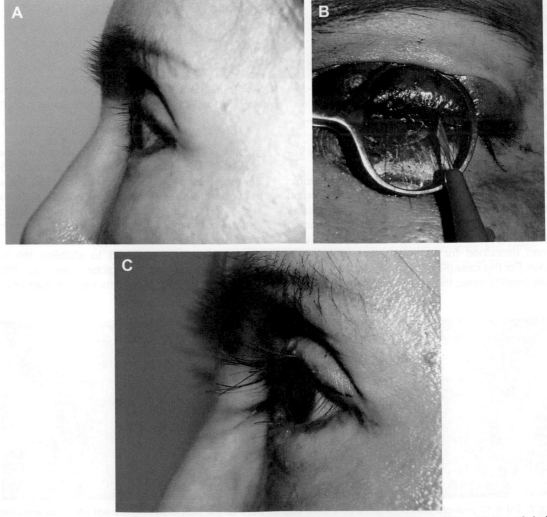

Fig. 9. (*A*) A 42-year-old woman with madarosis following a domestic hot oil kitchen accident. (*B*) Use of chalazion clamp and 22.5° Sharpoint blade is demonstrated. (*C*) One year after placement of 32 follicular unit grafts.

jeweler's forceps. Obtaining optimal direction of hair growth and curl as well as a good density are particularly difficult in this area, and it is important to leave the donor hair slightly longer to facilitate accurate directional placement.

SUMMARY

The use of hair transplantation in the camouflage of scarring alopecia can be a powerful tool in changing the lives of patients. We are all touched by the improvements we can make in the lives of others. Recently a letter from a patient who underwent multiple surgeries in the repair of extensive scarring alopecia from a bear mauling drove this point home. "…From your perspective…it's another day at the office. From my perspective-…it's a miracle. I am elated (and relieved) to know that when my hair grows back in, I will look like a 23-year-old woman again and not a disfigured 'bear-attack victim.' The results are stunning and even moved my fiancé to tears." The techniques used in restoring facial scars are still in a stage of evolution, and it is patients like this who inspire us to continue to work toward techniques and results that allow these patients to resume living happy, healthy, and productive lives.

The field of hair restoration surgery is a fascinating one. A tremendous amount has been learned over the years, and the field continues to change to better serve patients. Although there are many approaches that will ultimately result in a successful outcome, there are a few principles that should always be applied when approaching the camouflage of scars in the head and neck using hair grafts.

- Listen to your patients; what are their goals and are they realistic? Is hair grafting the best approach for their case?
- Play close attention to recipient incision density and direction.
- Carefully consider the vascular supply of the recipient bed.
- It is always better to graft conservatively and perform a staged second or third procedure rather than risking poor graft survival and wasting of a limited donor reservoir.
- When grafting the scalp, consider the patient's hairstyle and weigh graft placement to create the illusion of more density in cosmetically important areas when necessary.
- Always mimic nature, including creating irregularity and transitioning to larger hair grafts at the border between hair-bearing and non–hair-bearing skin.

When applying these techniques, the use of hair grafting is very safe and predictable, and can create a natural restoration for patients. Hair transplantation for the repair of complex scarring in the head and neck region is an accepted standard of care, and should be recognized as a critical component in restoring patients to their premorbid state.

REFERENCES

1. Nordstrom RE. Punch hair grafting under split-skin grafts on scalps. Plast Reconstr Surg 1979;64:1.
2. Headington JT. Transverse microscopic anatomy of the human scalp. Arch Dermatol 1984;120:449.
3. Bernstein RM, Rassmant WR, Szaniawki W, et al. Follicular transplantation. Int J Aesthet Restor Surg 1995;3:119–32.
4. Nakatsui T, Wong J, Groot D. Survival of densely packed follicular unit grafts using the lateral slit technique. Dermatol Surg 2008;34:1016–22.
5. Beehner M. Hairline design in hair replacement surgery. Facial Plast Surg 2008;24:389–403.
6. Nusbaum BP, Fuentefria S. Naturally occurring female hairline patterns. Dermatol Surg 2009;35:907–13.
7. Shapiro R. Principles and techniques used to create a natural hairline in surgical hair restoration. Facial Plast Surg Clin North Am 2004;12:201–17.
8. Ziering C, Krenitsky G. The Ziering whorl classification of scalp hair. Dermatol Surg 2003;29:817–21.
9. Bernstein RM, Rassman WR. Follicular transplantation. Dermatol Surg 1997;23:771–84.
10. Rassman WR, Bernstein RM. Follicular unit extraction: minimally invasive surgery for hair transplantation. Dermatol Surg 2002;28:720–8.
11. Poswal A. The preshaving protocol in body hair-to-scalp transplant to identify hair in anagen phase. Indian J Dermatol 2010;55:50–2.
12. Limmer BL. Micrograft survival. In: Stough DB, editor. Hair transplantation. 2nd edition. New York: Dekker; 1988. p. 310–6.
13. Cooley JE. Ischemia-reperfusion injury and graft storage solutions. Hair Transpl Forum Int 2004; 14(4):121.
14. Hwang S, Youn Kim Ho, Kim JC, et al. Recipient-site influence in hair transplantation: a confirmative study. Dermatol Surg 2009;35:1011–4.
15. Straub MP. Replacing facial hair. Facial Plast Surg 2008;24:446–52.
16. Wang J, Fan J, Chai J. Aesthetic eyelash elongation for Asians using a dense-packing single-hair grafting technique. Dermatol Surg 2010;36:1155–60.
17. Seyhan A, Yoleri L, Barutcu A. Immediate hair transplantation into a newly closed wound to conceal the final scar on hair-bearing skin. Plast Reconstr Surg 2000;105:5.
18. Barrera A. The use of micrografts and minigrafts for the treatment of burn alopecia. Plast Reconstr Surg 1999;103(2):581–4.

19. Barrera A. The use of micrografts and minigrafts in the aesthetic reconstruction of the face and scalp. Plast Reconstr Surg 2003;112(3):883–90.

20. Unger W, Nordstrom R. Hair transplantation under split-thickness skin grafts and very thin skin. In: Unger W, editor. Hair transplantation. 3rd edition. New York: Marcel Dekker; 1995. p. 312–7.

21. Jones R. Transplanting hair follicles into scar tissue and grafted skin. Presentation at International Society of Hair Restoration Surgery. Boston, October 23, 2010.

22. Klinger M, Marrazzi M, Vigo D. Fat injection for cases of severe burn outcomes: a new perspective of scar remodeling and reduction. Aesthetic Plast Surg 2008;32(3):465–9.

23. Emsen IM. The use of micrografts and minigrafts together with advancement of temporalis fascia and its periosteum on the treatment of burn alopecia. J Craniofac Surg 2008;19(4):907–9.

24. Blackwel KE, Rawnsley JD. Aesthetic considerations in scalp reconstruction. Facial Plast Surg 2008;24: 11–21.

25. Barrera A. The use of micrografts and minigrafts for the correction of postrhytidectomy lost sideburn. Plast Reconstr Surg 1998;102(6):2237–9.

26. Barrera A. Correcting retroauricular hairline deformity after face lift. Aesthet Surg J 2004;24(2):176–8.

27. Kilic A, Kilic A, Ilteris ME, et al. Lip scars camouflaged using microhair transplantation on male patients. Plast Reconstr Surg 2000;106(6):1340–1.

Index

Facial Plast Surg Clin N Am 19 (2011) 569–576
doi:10.1016/S1064-7406(11)00103-9

Moving?

Make sure your subscription moves with you!

To notify us of your new address, find your **Clinics Account Number** (located on your mailing label above your name), and contact customer service at:

Email: journalscustomerservice-usa@elsevier.com

800-654-2452 (subscribers in the U.S. & Canada)
314-447-8871 (subscribers outside of the U.S. & Canada)

Fax number: 314-447-8029

Elsevier Health Sciences Division
Subscription Customer Service
3251 Riverport Lane
Maryland Heights, MO 63043

ELSEVIER

Moving?

Make sure your subscription moves with you!

To notify us of your new address, find your Clinics Account Number (located on your mailing label above your name), and contact customer service at:

Email: journalscustomerservice-usa@elsevier.com

800-654-2452 (subscribers in the U.S. & Canada)
314-447-8871 (subscribers outside of the U.S. & Canada)

Fax number: 314-447-8029

Elsevier Health Sciences Division
Subscription Customer Service
3251 Riverport Lane
Maryland Heights, MO 63043

To ensure uninterrupted delivery of your subscription,
please notify us at least 4 weeks in advance of move.

Printed and bound by CPI Group (UK) Ltd, Croydon, CR0 4YY

03/10/2024

01040351-0009